Youth Renewed

*A Common Sense Approach to
Vibrant Health ... At Any Age*

by Bill Code, MD
and
Claudia Tiefisher

Cartoons by Jordan Rynierse
Cover Photograph © Tony Stone Images, Charles Krebs

The Chameleon Health Series Library
Chameleon Publishing, Canada

Published in Canada by
Chameleon Publishing & Graphics Ltd.
Calgary, AB

Canadian Cataloguing in Publication Data:

William E. Code, MD, FRCPC
Claudia Tiefisher
[Youth Renewed]
A Common Sense Approach to Vibrant Health ... at Any Age
Includes index.
ISBN 0-9687668-0-3
1. Emu Oil 2. Health 3. Weight Loss 4. Skin Care—Natural 5. Longevity
6. Nutrition 7. Essential Fatty Acids 8. Skin Conditions—Natural Remedies
Title:
        Youth Renewed
        A Common Sense Approach to Vibrant Health ... at Any Age

        Interior & Cover Design and Typesetting & Indexing
            by Chameleon Publishing & Graphics Ltd.
                Calgary, Alberta, Canada

        PRINTED IN CANADA

ACKNOWLEDGEMENTS

The authors would like to thank the following people, without whom this book could not have been possible:

The Codes—Alice, Denise, Laura, Brian and Warren.
A special thanks to Jeffrey Johns, recently deceased, who was instrumental in setting the international standards for emu oil. Thanks also to the International Emu Oil Standards Team. Heartfelt thanks for the support and help of Gordon Tiefisher and Doris and Wolfgang Hoehne.

"Everything which a man is depends on what he puts inside him."

— *Mark Twain*

CONTENTS

INTRODUCTION

An Entirely New Way to Look at Energy, Health and Longevity

Our lifestyles and our environment have caught up to us and indeed overtaken us on the road of life. We are not keeping up anymore. We have made life so fast, so impossibly fast, that it has left our bodies exhausted. The reason why is that just one hundred years ago, life was considerably different than it is today, and bodies—physiologically speaking—do not adapt and evolve that quickly. We lived life at a considerably slower pace. We had none of the "modern conveniences" we have today, but instead relied on manual labour. We did not live today's sedentary lifestyle. We did not rely on "quick and easy convenience" foods to help get us through our day. We did not have the machines and cars and chemicals polluting our environment.

In many ways, of course, life was much more difficult. Washing machines, central heating, telephones, and refrigerators are just a few of the modern conveniences few of us would want to do without. Medical science has made it possible for us to live longer, but we have to ask: are we healthier? It depends. If we managed to avoid diseases that were common 100 years ago, we were probably healthier then. If we didn't, we died young—polio, a bad flu or fever, diabetes—were all diseases for which we had no answers. A few years before that we didn't even know what caused flus and fevers. We didn't know how to properly handle food or dispose of our waste in order to minimize disease. In many countries around the world, this knowledge is still foreign.

It seems as though the price we pay for our knowledge on how to prevent and combat disease is a higher incidence of disease. The chemicals, machines, fuels, paper, computer systems, and man-hours that go into the research of the treatment of disease and the search for cures is putting such a strain on our environment (and on us), that the flip side of the coin is more and more disease. We are in a race with ourselves.

Are we keeping up? No. Statistics tell us that we have lost the war on cancer (though the diagnostic machine manufacturers and drug companies would have us believe differently), we still do not have an effective way to combat AIDS, and forget about bringing safe water and sufficient food to people all over the planet.

If you are hoping this book will have the answers to some of these questions, we offer you instead a point of departure, a way to begin to think about life differently, so that disease prevention is within your own personal grasp. We will offer you a clear and concise roadmap to living your life in a sane, rational, healthy way. We will describe in just enough detail exactly how your body works and why it sometimes breaks down. Far from being a medical journal, however, you will find an easy-to-digest, easy-to-understand guide that will illuminate why reaching for an apple is so much better than reaching for a donut (even though you may already know exactly why).

Imagine a machine like the engine of your car. It requires gas, air, oil, water, sparks, etc., all in the correct proportion, and all at the correct times, in order to run properly. Take any of those things away, or disturb their balance, and your engine will either seize, stall, overheat, or perform sluggishly.

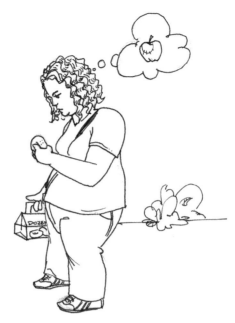

The way your body functions is similar, though far more complex. Your body needs air, food, water, nutrients, movement, stimulation, etc., in order to run optimally. Take any one of these away and you end up with a body functioning at below optimum or diseased. In the same way that adding sugar to your gas tank will destroy your car, consuming tobacco, excessive alcohol, drugs, or large amounts of a myriad of foods, or being constantly stressed, will damage certain pathways in your body and slowly destroy your health.

In the popular literature of the last 20 years, we have determined that we are an overweight, even somewhat obese, society, and that this condition is leading to so many of the diseases that are prevalent today (heart disease, stroke, diabetes, certain forms of cancer). The reasons for the obesity are our sedentary lifestyle and all the calories we eat, particularly those in simple carbohydrates, excessive saturated fats (bacon), and trans fats (hard margarine and convenience foods). In response to this, food manufacturers have created "lite", "low fat" and "no fat" versions of virtually everything. Duped into believing we can eat as much of this food as we want, we have ended up consuming far too many calories and are actually heavier on average than we were 20 years ago. The problem was the same 20 years ago as it is today: we consume too many calories, and, when we eat fat, it is the wrong kind. That, in a nutshell, is why so many of us are still overweight. Add to this the aggressive marketing of high calorie, high bad-fat food and increasingly inactive lifestyles thanks to things like computer games and the internet (the apparent popularity of jogging and health clubs notwithstanding), and you have a perfect recipe for a society with a chronic weight problem.

There exists such a simple recipe for good health. Yes, it requires time, commitment and consistency, but it is not difficult to grasp how it can be done. It is not *easy* to accomplish, but, when viewed with common sense and understanding, it is unbelievably *simple*. One need only adopt the principles and stick with them.

Youth Renewed

PROLOGUE

A Personal Introductory Word from Dr. Bill Code

WHERE WERE YOU AT AGE 42? WHERE DO YOU EXPECT TO BE? I'd like to describe what happened to me the final few days of my work.

As you'll note later in the book, I am a retired anaesthesiologist. This all came to pass in the summer of 1996, just before my 43rd birthday. I had noticed that there were problems with the needles I was using in my operating room and pain relief work. I'd contacted the supplier and they'd said, "No problem, Dr. Code, we'll send you out some more needles. There must be a problem with this batch." However, when I received the replacements, they were no better.

In my final week of work in August, before starting a couple of weeks of holiday, I noticed that I was having increasing problems emptying the syringe. Typically we start an anaesthetic case by emptying a 20 cc syringe with the right hand, injecting it into free-flowing intravenous tubing. However, by that final week, I was noticing that I needed two hands—one to hold the syringe and the other to push down the plunger. I am right-handed, and it was my right hand which was decidedly weaker. But my holidays were starting soon and I hoped that whatever the problem was, it would soon be relieved. As noted before, I was 42 years of age, and I had a sudden feeling that I was aging very, very quickly. Suddenly I became acutely interested in what I could do to renew or regain my so-called youth.

In the two months preceding this episode, I had noticed that while riding my bicycle to work, my right foot slipped off the pedal much too often. I worried that this would result in my having a minor (or major) crash. So, for the last two or three weeks of work, I had already quit riding the bicycle and was driving my car because I'd become worried about falling. The other subtle sign that I'd noticed was that at times my right foot would slap when I walked. People call this "foot drop", meaning that unless you consciously think of it, the affected foot will flop on the floor. I was curious why this was happening to me. I had follow-ups with my family doctor and then eventually with a neurologist at the University of British Columbia.

The neurologist advised I take six months off. I certainly had a neurological problem, and rest was the only known way to give the neurologic system the chance to heal and recover.

During this time of rest, I noticed an increasing number of symptoms and signs. Two magnetic resonance imaging (MRI) diagnostics were performed, and I was initially diagnosed with multiple sclerosis (MS).

Suddenly, I was faced with a chronic illness, with little resolution anticipated. The only recommended therapy was rest. This was astonishing and frightening. I had graduated from medical school some 18 years prior, done four years of general practice, including general practice anaesthesia and obstetrics. Following that I'd returned and studied five years of anaesthesia, including two years of research on the brain and how anaesthetics worked on the brain. After all this, I was now faced with being unable to practice.

In my entire medical career to that point, I had never looked intimately at the thought of having a chronic illness. I'd seen a large number of pain patients in my personal practice and attended many conferences regarding pain issues and other chronic problems. However, it was very different to now be on the inside looking out. I felt frustration, anger, and even a tendency towards loss of hope.

In the first few months, I discovered that I was not really recovering to any great degree. In follow-ups with my family doctor and neurologist, they suggested I plan a further six months off.

The time off had already caused a huge upheaval in my life—affecting my family, finances and, of course, myself personally. And I was learning that almost all adjustments to chronic illness happen in the first year.

I found myself looking at how to renew my youth, how to recover where I'd been. I had not anticipated having to leave the workforce in my early 40's. My personal journey with chronic illness had begun.

In November 1997, some 15 months after leaving "for my two-week holiday," I began to accept I wasn't going to get back to anaesthesia. My sister in Calgary (who also has MS), told me of a Vancouver conference on Complementary Choices in Medicine for people with MS. It was an important event. I met some people on their own journey who have helped me on mine.

This book will teach you some of what I have learned to help chronically ill people "renew their youth". Each chapter holds clues that might help you, the way they helped me. There are no "magic bullets" or drugs. There is some ancient and natural wisdom to be followed. Hopefully, my story will guide you on your own journey of health so that your epilogue is cheerier than your starting point.

Mine is.

CHAPTER 1

Fats & Fatty Acids or The Good, the Damaged & the Damaging

This book, as the title *Youth Renewed* suggests, will offer a blueprint to regaining youthful health and exuberance—a way to understand the possibility of drinking from the fountain of youth. Understand that there is no one answer, no one magic cure, no pill, potion or lotion that will take you there.

Many of our ills stem from consuming the wrong type of fat. It isn't just that we're eating too much fat (though we certainly are). It is also that we're not getting enough essential fatty acids (EFAs). They are called essential because we must get them from our diet; our bodies cannot manufacture them. This is a double-edged sword, and the vast majority of the population is being cut with it on both sides. It is the body's fight with bad fat and its being starved of good fat that are central to many of our health complaints—minor and major. It is critical to understand this, because it is both syndromes—too much damaged fat and a deficiency in good fat—that weaken all our cells and cell components. This in turn weakens organs and eventually the immune system (or makes it work overtime, causing it to turn on healthy tissues), and lays the groundwork for most of today's diseases.

The popular media has been obsessed with reporting how we eat too much fat and how it contributes to many diseases (which is, nonetheless, true). Although so many foods can now be obtained in "lite", "low fat" or "no fat" versions, we are heavier now, on average, than we were 20 years ago. The distinction that is *never* made in the 30-second commercials that pass for nutritional education for many people, is the distinction between good and damaged fat. Fats are not that complicated, but the science of fats has never properly been explained to most of us. Meanwhile, we take our knowledge base from "food" manufacturers. Their top priority is to take inexpensive ingredients that have a *long shelf life* and convince us that they are not only good for us, but that consuming these non-foods will also make us happier, richer, smarter and more popular. We must remember that the pizza, pudding, pie, and fast food manufacturers are just that: *manufacturers*. Modern processing methods have made it possible to buy food and set it on our shelves for months without it going rancid. We should be aware of the process that makes this possible in the first place.

Understanding Fats

Our bodies are chemical factories and chemical entities. That's why, when you hear someone complaining that something has a "chemical" smell, it's rather a non-sensical statement, though we all know what the person means. Though we are biological entities in that we reproduce and evolve, what makes the biology possible are the hundreds of thousands of chemical reactions that take place inside our bodies (and some on the outside) on an ongoing basis.

The smallest component within us is the atom. Groups of atoms bound together in a certain pattern make molecules. An example of a molecule would be a fat, protein, or carbohydrate molecule. Every molecule in *biology* (think back to your high school science class) contains carbon or is said to be carbon-based. What this means in practical terms is that it has the ability to burn; that is, it has energy and therefore has life. It is the way in which atoms (for example, in humans, nitrogen, carbon, oxygen, hydrogen) are grouped—*their arrangement*—that determines the kind of molecule they are. Atoms can be in long chains or short ones. They can be clustered together or shaped like a pyramid.

A molecule of any liquid oil or solid fat is made up of one molecule of glycerol (as in glycerin soap) to which one, two, or three fatty acid molecules are attached. The oil or fat is then referred to as a *mono*glyceride, *di*glyceride, or *tri*glyceride. Fatty acids are the building blocks of all fats and oils, both in our bodies and in our food. They come in a variety of shapes and sizes and are the main component of *triglycerides*, a bundle of molecules consisting mostly of fats, and the form in which fats are transported and stored in the body.

Fatty acids are groups of hydrogen, carbon, and oxygen atoms whose shapes resemble caterpillars—complete with heads. The

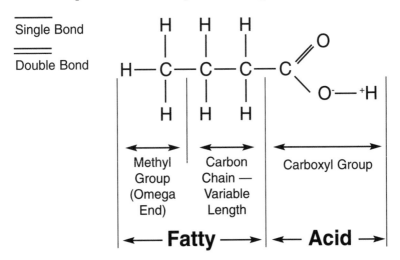

Figure 1-1: A basic fatty acid structure.
This one is saturated.

"head" end of the molecule is the "carboxyl" part (also known as the acid group and is the end that contains the oxygen atoms). The "body" is the fatty chain, made up of carbon and hydrogen in different configurations, and of varying lengths *(see figure 1-1)*[1]. The longer the fatty chain (the number of atoms before you get to the "head"[2]—made up of a carbon-hydrogen chain), the more difficult it is for the human body to digest.

Types of Fatty Acids

You hear all the time about saturated and unsaturated fats. You also hear about *mono*unsaturated and *poly*unsaturated fats. But do you know what they mean, beyond a vague understanding that one may be better for you than the other?

Basically, there are three categories of fatty acids: *saturated fatty acids, monounsaturated fatty acids,* and *polyunsaturated fatty acids.* Each of the three categories of fatty acids is defined by the type of bond between the carbon atoms in the chain. As you recall from *figure 1-1,* a basic fatty acid structure is made up of a chain of carbon atoms joined together. The number of carbon atoms in the chain and the types of bonds between carbon atoms determines the particular fatty acid.

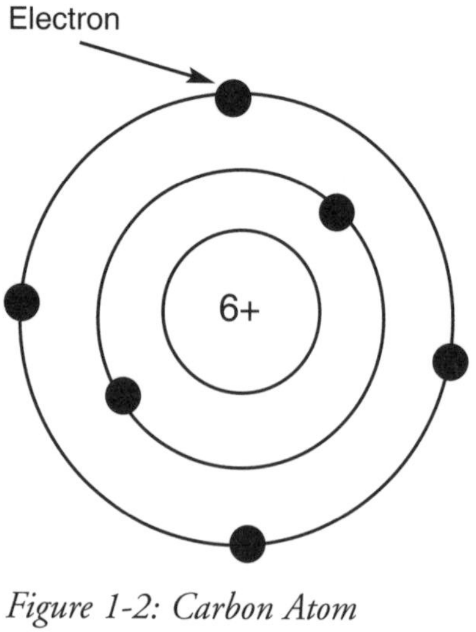

A carbon atom has four electrons in its outer ring *(see figure 1-2).* It wants to pair each electron with an electron from some other atom. When carbon shares an electron with another atom, such as hydrogen, each pair of shared electrons forms a single bond. Carbon can share its 4 electrons in this way: 2 electrons are paired with 2

Figure 1-2: *Carbon Atom*

electrons from 2 hydrogen atoms and the 2 remaining electrons are paired with electrons from 2 other carbon atoms *(see figure 1-3)*. The resulting bonds between the carbon atoms are thus single bonds.

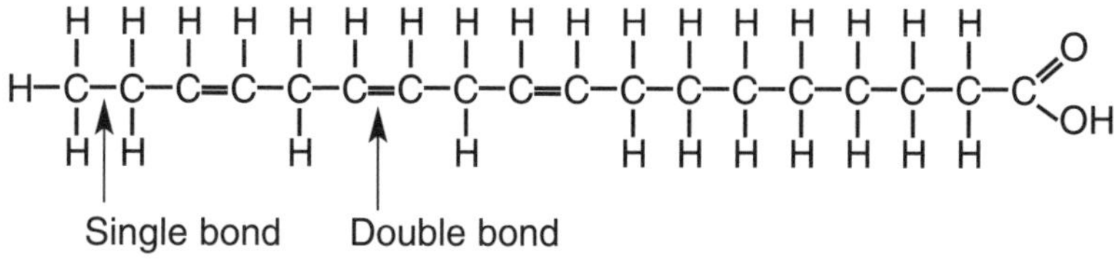

Figure 1-3: Alpha-Linolenic Acid (ALA)

Carbon can also pair its 4 electrons this way: 1 electron is paired with 1 hydrogen atom, 1 electron is paired with 1 carbon atom, and its 2 remaining electrons are paired with 2 electrons from a single carbon atom (remember that carbon has a total of 4 electrons to share). When one carbon atom shares two electrons with another carbon atom in this way, a double bond is formed.

Double bonds are unstable and can easily be broken. Food manufacturers break them by bubbling hydrogen through the fat in a process called *hydrogenation*. When the double bond ruptures, an electron is left floating around, not attached to anything. Electrons don't like this. They hate a *vacuum* (being *unattached)* and so search frantically for something to attach to. What they attach to is hydrogen, and single bonds are formed between carbon atoms *(see figure 1-4)*.

As mentioned above, fatty acids are categorized by the type of bond between carbon atoms in the carbon chain. In saturated fatty acids, all the carbon atoms are joined by single bonds. When this occurs, the fatty acid has the most number of hydrogen atoms it can have attached to the carbon atoms in the chain. It is therefore "saturated" with hydrogen. Saturated fats are usu-

Broken double bond

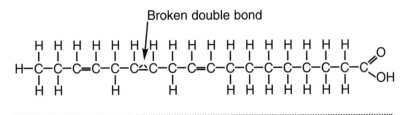

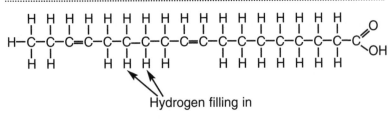

Hydrogen filling in

Figure 1-4: The process of hydrogenation or simply heating a liquid oil such as canola causes double bonds to break. Unattached carbon electrons latch onto hydrogen until all electrons are bonded.

ally solid or semi-solid at room temperature. Examples of saturated fats include butterfat, animal fat, coconut oil, palm oil, and palm kernel oil.

Monounsaturated fats have one *(mono)* double bond in the fatty acid chain. Olive oil, canola oil, high-oleic safflower, and high-oleic sunflower oil are all monounsaturated fats. They are liquid at room temperature. At colder temperatures, they become cloudy or semi-solid. Try putting olive oil in the refrigerator and you will see it become white in colour and solid.

Polyunsaturated fats have two or more double bonds between carbon atoms, hence the designation *poly*. Polyunsaturated fats are liquid at room temperature and include corn oil, safflower oil, soybean oil, flaxseed oil, primrose oil, borage oil, walnut oil, and grapeseed oil. Double bonds can occur between any two carbon atoms in a carbon chain.

Polyunsaturated oils can be hardened by agitation, heating, or hydrogenation. When polyunsaturated fatty acids are agitated or heated (as in using corn oil for your chicken stir fry), the double bonds break. It doesn't take much heat to do this. Even vigorous stirring can rupture double bonds. When a double bond is ruptured during hydrogenation, hydrogen fills the gap and the oil becomes saturated. This is how we turn a polyunsaturated fatty acid (like that found in liquid soybean or corn oil) into a saturated fatty acid. This saturation with hydrogen causes the liquid oil to become solid at room temperature and increases shelf life by many weeks or even months. Saturated fats are much slower to go rancid, hence their longer shelf life.

If you read the label on the side of a jar of margarine, peanut butter, granola bar, packaged cookies, or cake mix, you will usually see the ingredients: *hydrogenated corn oil* or *hydrogenated peanut oil* or *hydgogenated canola oil* or *hydrogenated vegetable oil*. The process that the fats undergo to become *hydrogenated*—the process which turns them from a liquid oil into a solid fat—you now understand.

A consequence of hydrogenation is the formation of *trans* fatty acids or *damaged fats*. Polyunsaturated fats become trans fats even if only one of their double bonds is hydrogenated. Trans fats have a molecular structure that the human body does not know what to do with. These fats, now damaged (even with one double bond broken), may fool the body by the resemblance they bear to *undamaged* polyunsaturated fatty acids. This is particularly dangerous as the body may use them in the manufacture of enzymes, hormones, and cell walls.

Because the body doesn't know what to do with the trans fats—as you'll read more about in Chapter 2—it often dumps them into bile or into arteries, where they may become the start of *atherosclerotic plaques*. The presence of these plaques in our arteries is one of the primary indicators for increased risk in developing heart disease.

Trans and saturated fats are very stable, whereas unsaturated fats are less stable. The human body is designed to use unsaturated fatty acids by taking their molecular structure and pairing them with the molecular structure of other tissues in the body. This creates each of our trillions of cells—including our brain cells (walls and interior structures), as well as enzymes, hormones, and other body tissues. As with animals, we also take those double bond fatty acid molecules and convert them into different types of molecules—building blocks—that the body needs for correct growth and function. The fact that unsaturated fats are unstable is important and desirable. Without their ability to alter their form, marrying up with other molecules to build new things, what good would they be to us as building blocks? Please consider trans or damaged fats as especially confusing for our bodies as they may look almost correct, but do not function well once into a cell wall.

This is so important to understand. These unsaturated fatty acids, especially the omega-3 and to some extent the omega-6, are required (they are *essential)* to the manufacture of life-dependent, health-dependent cells in the human body. It is the molecular structure of these fatty acids that is so desirable, not the fact that they are simply fats (as you must by now understand). The longer-chained, more stable, hard, *saturated* fats, are the ones the body prefers to use for energy. However, if the essential fatty acids' primary purpose has been fulfilled, then the EFAs can also be used for energy. Remember, too, from the point of view of weight maintenance, the body takes fatty acids, stores them in the body, and *then* uses them for energy purposes. Carbohydrates are used more directly for energy. Keep in mind, though, that the body often makes new fat from carbohydrates, especially if the liver and EFAs are not in ideal balance.

So, damaged fats experience a what-good-are-they response when they enter our bodies. Because they are hard, stable, and unyielding, the body cannot break them down or do anything with them. The body responds by storing them in fat deposit tissues around the body (belly, thighs, upper arms, etc.) and also around organs and *in* organs, such as your liver. Saturated fats, in excess, will cause similar problems, but they are not *nearly* as damaging as trans fats.

Usability of Fatty Acids

As mentioned previously, all fats and oils are comprised of molecules that are shaped somewhat like caterpillars *(see figure 1-5)*[3]. Fatty acid molecules occurring in nature construct their double bonds in what is called a *cis* configuration. What this means is that wherever the double bond is situated, the hydrogen atoms linked to the carbon atoms are always linked on the same side *(see*

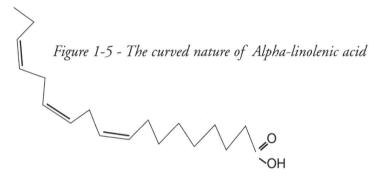

Figure 1-5 - The curved nature of Alpha-linolenic acid

figure 1-6). The hydrogen atoms repel one another and the fatty acid chain kinks to take up some of the space opposite the hydrogen atoms. When this same molecule is hydrogenated, one double bond is broken and hydrogen atoms are placed on *the other* side of the chain as well, so that you end up with an *unkinked* or straightened out caterpillar *(see figure 1-7)*[4]. Hence, once one double bond is hydrogenated, the other unsaturated double bonds can confuse the body into using this trans molecule. This can stiffen cell walls and interfere with cell and organ functions.

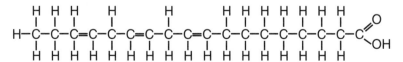

Figure 1-6 - Alpha-Linolenic Acid

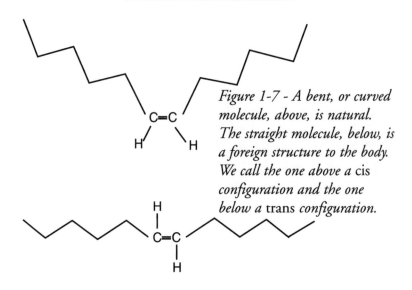

Figure 1-7 - A bent, or curved molecule, above, is natural. The straight molecule, below, is a foreign structure to the body. We call the one above a cis *configuration and the one below a* trans *configuration.*

The molecules that make our cells are not designed to fit with these straight molecules—they are curved, twisted (think of a double stranded helix, like DNA), and kinked also.

Interestingly, when cooking with high heats, butter is better as it is a saturated fat, so there is no trans element to confuse the body. Butter is constructed of butyric acid—one of the shortest saturated fatty acid molecules, and relatively healthy for you, when used in moderation.

If you are going to eat deep-fried foods, tallow (beef fat) is better than canola or other vegetable oils.

Think of the molecules in your body as a lock and digested food as the key. When you take foods into your body, if the molecules that make up the foods occur naturally (that is, they have not been tampered with in any way) the digested food will fit neatly into the lock. If we try to insert a key that doesn't fit, the key is simply rejected. If you carry this analogy along, you can see that an excess of trans fats (*by far* the worst type of fat) will have a negative effect on your body. We were certainly better off 50 years ago—even in the 60's in North America—when fats were polyunsaturated (PUFAs), monounsaturated (MUFAs), or saturated—before we ever heard of trans fats and hydrogenation.

Take for example your brain. The cells in your brain are composed of about 50 per cent fat. *If you consume plenty of essential fatty acids in your diet, you are providing your brain with exactly the building blocks it needs. This results in clearer thinking, increased alertness, and a heightened ability to focus and concentrate. It will literally make you smarter!*

If you eat too much saturated fat and trans fat, here's what occurs in your body. Your liver is the main fat burning and metabolizing engine of your body. A lifetime of excess amounts of damaged fats makes for an overworked liver. This means that not only do you not properly process fats you consume, but your liver actually begins to store them, somewhere in your body. However, if the body lacks enough insulin, the fats become triglycerides and are now preferentially stored in the liver itself (similar to excess alcohol and fatty liver)[5]. Thankfully, it is for the most part reversible with correct diet and exercise. In the meantime, though, this sluggish liver has a hard time processing toxins. When this happens and the liver becomes overloaded with toxins, fats, or undigested proteins, it in effect throws up its hands, gives up and dumps these toxins into your bile or directly into your bloodstream. Now you have these particles floating around in your bloodstream, going through your heart, and being dumped into arteries and organs throughout your body. This greatly accelerates the aging process.

What happens when these toxins are dumped into the bloodstream? Your thinking will be foggy and cloudy and you will find it difficult to concentrate. The undigested proteins can trigger allergic reactions and, eventually, begin to set the stage for autoimmune disorders. Undigested fats are re-packaged and circulated in your bloodstream. This contributes to atherosclerosis, stroke, and heart disease. An excess of trans or damaged fats also paves the way for obesity.

Essential and Unsaturated Fatty Acids

Essential fatty acids (EFAs) are called "essential" for two reasons. One, because they are essential in the diet as the body cannot manufacture them, and two, because they are essential for health. Many people do double damage to their bodies with the common North American diet. They eat far, far too much of the damaging trans fats (found in margarine and most processed foods), and consume an excessive amount of saturated (animal) fats found in butter and other dairy products and in most meats. On top of this, most people do not eat nearly enough of the EFAs (found in flax seeds, most types of fish, dark green leafy vegetables, cold pressed oils, nuts, and seeds). Making matters worse, it is usually the presence of too much "bad" fat in the diet (and calories, which come from every source, including proteins and carbohydrates) which contributes to obesity or overweight. The response by the dieter is usually to attempt to cut all fat from the diet. But we're doing it all wrong.

Two things happen when we start cutting fat from our diet. First of all, we need calories to live, for energy, for cellular reproduction, for life. Our bodies will demand food and until we give it food—*and the right kind, that is nutritious*—we can expect to remain hungry and sluggish. What is the right kind of food? Whole food—not some processed composite of white flour, instant potatoes, or packaged macaroni dinner. If we are convinced *all* fats are evil, we will reach for carbohydrates for the simple reason that *we are hungry*. This is another double-edged sword. You will read more about this in the chapter on digestion. Unless we reach for the right type of carbohydrate (it should contain some fiber and for most people meals should contain *some* protein), we send our insulin levels skyrocketing. That signals our bodies to convert the sugar (the carbohydrate) into fat. Fiber, in effect, puts the brakes on the absorption of sugars we consume (as does protein), creating what might be called a *sustained release*. Once again, *whole foods* contain more fiber, vita-

Fatty Acids Made Simple

The Omega-6 Family

The Omega-3 Family

Linoleic Acid (LA)
(Found in vegetable oils, seeds and nuts.)

Alpha-Linolenic Acid (ALA)
(Found in green leafy vegetables, flax, flaxseed oil, canola oil, emu oil, walnuts, and Brazil nuts.)

Your body converts LA into:

⬇

Your body converts ALA into:

⬇

Gamma-Linolenic Acid (GLA)
(GLA is also found in borage and primrose oil.)

Eicosapentaenoic Acid (EPA)
(EPA is also found in fish oil.)

Your body converts GLA into:

⬇

Your body converts EPA into:

⬇

Arachidonic Acid (AA)
(AA is also found in meat.)

⬇

Docosahexaenoic Acid (DHA)
(DHA is also found in fish oil.)

⬇

The Omega-6 Family of Eicosanoids

The Omega-3 Family of Eicosanoids

Adapted from: The Omega Diet by A. Simopoulos, M.D. & J. Robinson, Harper Perennial, 1999, p. 40 mins, and other *phytochemicals* to help us.

Now, we will crave fats too, especially if we have made a concerted effort to cut them out. (Remember, *we need fats*.) So, what happens? Our bodies become so starved for *good* fats, and send out so many signals telling us we need fat, that we turn into the nearest drive-through and load up on heavy combinations of trans fats and saturated fats. Nowhere in the world will you find a drive-through menu, take-out, or convenience food high in essential fatty acids. Even worse, these foods are also high in simple carbohydrates (white buns) and low in fiber (unless you're having a side salad, which contains far less fiber and food value than you might believe, considering some of the ingredients and the fatty dressings likely to be poured on top). The meat is fatty, fried and has no fiber.

We need good fats. We need essential fatty acids like we need the sunshine and the rain. This cannot be over-emphasized, and the more natural and pure the source, the better. Limiting intake of damaged fats is important, but even more important is to make sure you are getting enough essential fatty acids in your diet. If you aren't getting enough, you need to take supplements.

There are many reasons for this: first, not getting enough good fat signals your body that you are starving. That slows down metabolism. If the body continues to receive these signals—that it is never going to get enough food to satisfy itself—then it will continue to use what it gets sparingly, i.e., it will burn calories slowly, and store what it can (as fat) for future use.

Essential fatty acids are normal components of the walls of our cells. Without sufficient EFAs our cell walls and the cell's internal structures develop holes and become prone to leakage and poor energy transfer. EFAs also enable the cell membrane to eliminate toxins from the inside to the outside of the cell and especially to allow liver cells to cleanse the blood of toxic material. EFAs keep your cell barriers strong and thus improve the efficiency of your immune system.

Adequate EFAs in your diet have desirable effects on many disorders. They improve skin and hair, reduce blood pressure, aid in the prevention of arthritis, lower cholesterol and triglyceride levels, and reduce the risk of blood clot formation. They are beneficial for candida yeast conditions, cardiovascular disease, eczema, and psoriasis. Found in high concentrations in the brain (especially the omega-3 group), EFAs aid in the transmission of nerve impulses and are needed for the normal development and functioning of the brain. A deficiency of essential fatty acids can lead to an impaired ability to learn and recall information. A deficiency has even been associated with attention-deficit hyperactivity disorder (ADHD). So, consider this: the next time you are called a "fathead", it is really a compliment!

There are two essential fatty acids: omega-3 and omega-6 fatty acids. They are named "3" and "6", respectively, because in the carbon chain described earlier, there is a double bond between the carbon atoms between the third and fourth carbon atom in omega-3, and between the sixth and seventh carbon atom in omega-6 *(see figure 1-3)*. There may be more than one double bond in the chain—unsaturated fatty acids in nature have from one to six double bonded carbon atoms. Life forms manufacture certain types of fatty acids. Plants are capable of forming these double bonds close to the beginning of the carbon chain; humans are not.

An interesting note here: if animals, especially birds, are fed a diet high in EFAs, there will be more of these EFAs available for us in their eggs, meat, and fat—for example omega-3 chickens and emus.

The point to understand here is that we *need* the 3-position and 6-position fatty acids. These are the fatty acids the body prefers to use for the manufacture of enzymes and hormones, rather than for use as energy. The body prefers to use the longer chain saturated fatty acids for energy, for fuel. It can also take these fatty acids (the longer ones) and *de*saturate them, converting them to a form more preferable for enzyme and hormone manufacture. However, it cannot convert them into the form where the double bond appears in the 3 or 6 position. We must therefore get these fatty acids from our diets. The human body cannot make double bonds prior to the 7th carbon atom.

Unsaturated Omega-3 Family

• **Alpha-linolenic acid** (ALA), sometimes incorrectly called linolenic acid, is found in flax, hemp seed, canola, soy beans, and dark, green leafy vegetables. Flax seed is the best source—about 50 per cent of its fatty acid content is made up of ALA. As we've tried to make clear, this is the most important essential fatty acid[6] *(see figure 1-6)*. Why is it the most important? Because our current diets often provide enough omega-6—they are abundantly available in grain oils such as canola. Consequently, the balance between omega-3 and omega-6 is upset.

Excess omega-6 fatty acids (and a deficiency in omega-3 fatty acids) are being blamed for creating too many of the negative *eicosanoids* (you will read more about eicosanoids in Chapter 9). Seventy per cent of us need to increase our omega-3s by consuming Canadian flax, fish oils, and dark, leafy green vegetables.

Flax seeds and their oil are high in omega-3 EFAs, helping to restore the optimal balance of omega-3 to omega-6 in the diet. We get far more omega-6 from our diet than we do the omega-3. Flax seeds are an excellent source of omega-3.

• **Eicosapentaenoic acid** (EPA) and **Docosahexaenoic acid** (DHA) are found in the oils of cold water fish and marine animals. Salmon, trout, mackerel, sardines, and other cold water marine animals are rich sources, containing up to 30% combined EPA and DHA[7]. Our bodies can make both of these, as long as it has enough ALA.

Unsaturated Omega-6 Family

• **Linoleic acid** (LA) is found in safflower, sunflower, hemp, soybean, walnut, pumpkin, and sesame. Safflower and sunflower are the richest sources[8].

• **Gamma-linolenic acid** (GLA) can be found in the highest concentrations in borage oil and black currant seed oil, followed by evening primrose oil. Gamma-linolenic acid has attracted a lot of attention in the last few years as being an excellent remedy for premenstrual and menopausal conditions and their symptoms.

• **Dihomogamma-linolenic acid** (DGLA) is present in mothers' milk.

• **Arachidonic acid** (AA) is not found in peanut oil (see under Saturates family), contrary to the name's suggestion of this. It is found in meats and other animal products.

Monounsaturated Omega-9 Family

• **Oleic acid** (OA) is found in large quantities in olive, canola, almond, avocado, peanut, pecan, cashew, filbert, and macadamia oils. Land animal fats are other sources of OA. This is a fatty acid that is readily manufactured by the body[9].

Fats are classified as saturated, monounsaturated, or polyunsaturated according to the dominant fatty acid making up the fat. For example, olive oil is 70% oleic and emu is 55%. Therefore, these fats are mainly monounsaturated. Emu oil differs from olive oil—it has more omega-3 and omega-6 fatty acids than olive oil.

Monounsaturated Omega-7 Family

• **Palmitoleic acid** (POA) is found in tropical oils, especially coconut and palm kernel[10].

Saturated Family

The family of saturated acids has had a bad rap. They are much, much better for us than trans fats, especially the shorter saturated fatty acids found in butter.

• **Stearic acid** (SA) is found in high quantities in beef, mutton, pork, butter, and cocoa butter[11].

• **Palmitic acid** (PA) is in the tropical fats: coconut, palm, and palm kernel[12].

• **Butyric acid** (BA) is found in butter[13].

• **Arachidic acid** is present in peanuts[14].

Points & Tips

- It is vital to understand that essential fatty acid oils must be consumed in their original form—that is, once they are processed or over-heated, they become the trans fats you want to avoid;

- Avoid *hydrogenated* and *partially hydrogenated* vegetable oil products (again, trans fats)[15];

- When choosing oils, select cold pressed oils. Oils that are not cold pressed are extracted with a chemical called hexane. Hexane is highly effective, but may have adverse side effects if residual amounts remain in the oil;

- If you are using olive oil, spend the little extra money and buy virgin or extra virgin olive oil;

- Oils you purchase from the store should, if at all possible, be stored in a dark or opaque bottle. Light destroys the oil over time, especially omega-3s, which are much more fragile and unstable than omega-6s;

- Flax seed oil can not be heated at all without breaking double bonds;

- Ways to use flax oil: sprinkle it over your salads, or add a tablespoon to rice or vegetables *after cooking*; grind up organic flax seeds in a little coffee grinder and sprinkle over just about anything. Two tablespoons a day will give you lots of omega-3;

- Butter, in moderation, is better than hardened margarine made with hydrogenated or partially hydrogenated vegetable oil. Margarine should never pass your lips, especially if you are cooking it at high heats;

- If you spread something on your bread, try hummus (mashed chickpeas with garlic), olive oil, avocado with either a bit of lemon or, for a savory flavor, chopped green onions and pepper (it's addicting, delicious, and so good for you!);
- Snack on nuts (soy nuts are good!) and raw seeds like sunflower and pumpkin instead of chips.

Having said how important it is to avoid damaged fats and how equally important it is to find a way to incorporate good fats into your diet, don't go overboard. Good fats have as many calories as damaged fats (9 per gram). A good rule of thumb is, "when you eat fat, make sure it's good fat." You will get plenty of EFAs if you:

- Eat fish a few times a week (always steam or broil, never fry);
- Add ground up flax seeds to your diet daily;
- Eat plenty of raw, fresh, dark green leafy vegetables;
- Spread avocado on your bread. Avocados used to be called "poor man's" or "sailor's" butter because it was inexpensive, creamy, and didn't spoil on long ship voyages. You can mash ripe avocados or slice them thinly. Beware, though: a regular avocado contains about 35 grams of fat. Use in moderation;
- Take supplements which provide EFAs in various combinations. If you want to supplement, try Nature's Way Certified Organic Flax Seed Oil, Udo's Perfect Balance, or Omega Nutrition Flax Seed Oil, or any other organic flax or combination oil, available in health food stores;
- An excellent supplement to obtain some of the essential fatty acids is emu oil, which is much the same as olive oil, except with additional omega-3 and omega-6 fatty acids, and is available in capsule form. In the chapters that discuss emu oil's properties, you will read about this highly valuable nutrient source. Suffice it to say here that it may be the unique qualities of the various components naturally present in emu oil that have such beneficial effects.

This unique working together of different properties is sometimes known as "synergy." The dictionary definition of synergy is: *the interaction or co-operation of two or more agents or substances to produce an effect that exceeds or enhances the sum of their individual effects*. In other words, if you extracted the essential or active substances from something such as emu oil, and took them separately, they wouldn't have the same effect as if you took them all together in their original form. There are components in most natural products that haven't been identified yet. These components, or the unique way in which they interact with one another, or some unique relationship they have with one another, may be the very key that makes the product so effective. It is also difficult to get such a wide variety of essential fatty acids from any other single food or nutrient source. Please see the fatty acid composition of various foods in the appendix.

Once you get in the habit of healthy eating, and in particular paying attention to damaged fats and good fats, you will find such a huge difference in how you feel. Your energy level will go up, you will sleep better at night, you will be thinking more clearly, and you will be able to watch your weight drop. If you make eating like this part of your lifestyle, you will be able to maintain an ideal weight much more easily. Also, make sure you are getting plenty of vitamins (A, C, E, etc.) and minerals (such as calcium, magnesium), get lots of rest, and at least moderate, but regular, exercise for optimum health.

CHAPTER 2

A Tour of the Digestion System in your Body on a Typical Day

Have you ever considered what happens inside your body throughout a typical day? Have you wondered what effects digestion, or *indigestion*, have on your body? Indigestion makes you feel unwell, but is that all? Or does it have wider-ranging effects you haven't given much thought to? We'll answer these questions and also offer surprising, practical insight on this day-long tour.

We'll pick a working day, since, alas, most of us have more work days than play days. If you live in a temperate, not-too-northern climate, you'll be awakened by the sun, or at least by an increase of light in your bedroom. If you've had a full eight to ten hours sleep, you ought to wake feeling refreshed, rejuvenated, and ready to tackle the day. Chances are, though, you've had only five or six hours sleep. Those precious few hours may have been interrupted by trips to the bathroom, crying children, illness—a cold or one with chronic pain, a snoring partner or your own digestive system playing with your head. A system full of undigested food can make you wake suddenly, experience nightmares, or fail to allow you to drop into that deep "rapid-eye-movement" sleep that is so essential to well-being.

There's a lot you can do to ensure you get a good night's sleep … but that's ahead of where we are. It's morning. Your clock radio is bringing you news, traffic, and weather. You feel tense already because you know it's going to be a struggle to get to work on time—you have to get the kids off to school, pack lunches, and there's a report buried somewhere on the desk that you're supposed to give to your boss at 9:00 this morning. The traffic report says that your favourite route to the office is tied up due to an accident. You crack the venetian blinds and discover it's raining—again. You sigh and as you do so, you feel a faint tickle in the back of your throat that signals an oncoming cold or flu. And it's only Tuesday.

But life goes on and you're a trooper. Off to the kitchen to pour yourself the cup of coffee you set up on the automatic drip coffee maker the night before. If you're like many people, you can't get anything going without your morning cup of coffee. Coffee is a central nervous system stimulant. The brain, in response to this stimulation, signals the adrenal glands to produce more adrenalin. This all takes a while, of course—you don't feel the jolt immediately. When your body produces adrenalin in response to something other than fear (the primary reason your body releases this hormone), it has no reasonable place to use up the adrenalin it has released, and so it is reabsorbed. When you drink several cups of coffee throughout your day, you are continually putting your body through this surge of adrenalin and the after-effect slump, leaving you feeling exhausted.

In the olden days, when our lives were ruled by the sun, we went to bed after dark (shortly after), and rose with the sun. This makes sense and is how our bodies are designed to function. Now we live in a 24-hour world, and as soon as it's dark we flip on lights all around the house as needed. We work shift work, which is very damaging to the overall well-being of the body. We watch TV after dinner—dinner usually being a high fat and/or convenient concoction of semi-food. Meanwhile, our digestive

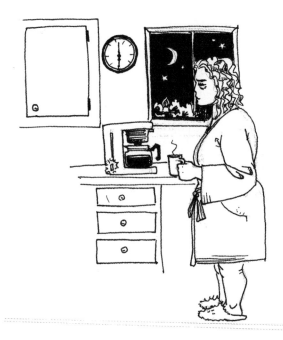

system labours under the load of food we have ingested, and our brain and the rest of our nervous system are stimulated by the flickering images on TV. What this stimulation does is decrease our body's cues to produce *melatonin*. This is the hormone that starts to be produced when it gets dark out, and which helps us sleep at night. While we sleep, *serotonin* is manufactured, and is then there to give us that kick-start out of bed early in the morning. Ironically, melatonin is manufactured from serotonin—one cannot be made without the presence of the other.

Okay, where were we? In the kitchen, sipping (or is that gulping?) coffee. The kids are getting up now, and you have to organize making lunches, taking a shower, having breakfast. Perhaps you are one of the smaller percentage of people who exercise in the morning, so your routine would also involve going out for a run, or maybe you pack your gear to the gym and have your morning shower there after your work-out. Morning exercise is very beneficial to your health, but exercising late in the morning—about 10:00 or 11:00—is ideal. Since this is not possible for most people whose working days run from 9 to 5 or thereabouts, early morning exercise is a good alternative.

Depending on your level of fitness and your exercise goals, you should have something to eat before you head to the gym or out for that run. Your body, upon waking, requires four things: fiber, fluid, food energy (*nutritious* calories), and vitamin C. Those are the four prongs upon which you should begin every day. They provide you with early energy to help get you through the day and will help you attain and maintain an ideal weight. Remember, if you starve yourself in an attempt to lose weight or if you skip meals due to stress or "busy-ness," you do yourself a grave injustice. The human body has been evolving for a blink of an eye, physiologically speaking, and we still remember very well how hard we had to fight for "valuable" food—proteins and fats—when we were hunter-gatherers. In response to days with very little food, our bodies adapted by slowing down metabolism. We could call it "the starvation response." This was smart as it conserved what little fuel we had available to us. The same thing still happens today. When you don't eat, your metabolism slows down and you burn *fewer* calories than you would if you ate at least three regular meals, preferably four to six smaller meals, spread throughout the day (also called grazing).

With all the knowledge we have about good health these days, we'll assume most of you won't eat a donut for breakfast. If you do, though, you will certainly get the energy rush you were looking for. However, it isn't sustained energy in any conceivable sense of the word. The donut is comprised of some *mildly* complex carbohydrates (the white flour), simple carbohydrates (the sugar), and trans fats. The uptake of the sugar is instantaneous as there is no fiber to slow this process down. Your body responds by making *insulin*, which signals your liver to make and store *glycogen* (glycogen is the stored form of *glucose*). Your liver can convert and store up to two-thirds of the sugars in a meal for later use. After it performs this function, if insulin levels are still high (insulin is created in response to sugars being ingested), the rest of the sugars in the meal will be converted to fatty acids, which are then packaged in preparation for transport to the fat deposit areas of the body. So you can see how sugar—especially simple sugars—contributes to excess fat.

Unfortunately, you're not much better off with a sourdough bagel. White flour items are quickly broken down to *glucose*—a simple sugar also known as a *monosaccharide*. Any white flour item, or any food high in simple carbohydrates like mashed potatoes and white pasta, that doesn't contain much *fiber*, is processed too quickly by the body. These items are high in *starch*. Though starch and fiber are both technically complex carbohydrates, they are not the same thing. This distinction is lost on many people. Fiber, no matter what form it comes in, is devoid of any vitamins or minerals and has no calories (because we don't digest it, though our helpful bacteria do). Even so, it is vital to our health.

A Short Discussion about Fiber

Fiber can be either soluble or insoluble. *Insoluble fiber* is the kind that our bodies cannot break down—in other words, we do not digest it. Insoluble fibers include *cellulose*—an indigestible carbohydrate found in the outer layer of vegetables and fruits. It is found in apples, beets, Brazil nuts, broccoli, carrots, celery, green beans, lima beans, pears, peas, and whole grains. Another indigestible fiber is *hemicellulose*, which absorbs water. This kind promotes weight loss, helps prevent colon cancer, and relieves constipation. It is found in apples, bananas, beans, beets, cabbage, corn, green leafy vegetables, pears, peppers, and whole grain cereals. A third common insoluble fiber is *lignin*, which is helpful in lowering *cholesterol* levels. It also aids in the prevention of the formation of gallstones by binding with bile acids and removing cholesterol before stones can form. Lignin is found in flax seeds[1], Brazil nuts (those Brazil nuts are *so* good for you!), carrots, green beans, peaches, peas, potatoes, strawberries, tomatoes, and whole grains.

Soluble fiber or *water-soluble fiber* is in the form of *pectins, gums,* and *mucilages.* These are found mainly in citrus fruits, apples, potatoes, dried peas and beans, oatmeal, and oat bran. Besides having a similar cholesterol-lowering effect as lignin, these types of fiber also help to stabilize *blood sugar levels.*

If you haven't been eating a lot of fiber in your diet, it is wise to increase intake slowly. Sudden increases in fiber consumption can result in cramping, diarrhea, and flatulence. If you are concerned about the level of fiber in your diet, take a top quality fiber supplement. The best ones contain oat bran and rice bran or psyllium seed. You can buy psyllium seed in bulk form from your health food store.

In a food high in carbohydrates, it is the ratio of carbohydrate to fiber which makes it a "good" or "bad" food. If the fiber is high, there is a good energy supply and a low potential for fat storage. If there is little or no fiber, the opposite is true. The higher the fiber, the more slowly the sugars or starches in the food will be absorbed into the bloodstream, giving you sustained energy release. There are numerous other benefits to this scenario. You will feel full longer with a hunk of whole grain bread or an apple than with a donut. You will be supplying your body with a host of essential nutrients in the form of vitamins, minerals, fats, phytochemicals, and proteins *along with* the carbohydrate and fiber. Phytochemicals are the biologically active substances in plants that are responsible for giving them color, flavour, and natural disease resistance. Some of these substances are known to fight cancer in humans. Whole foods—particularly fresh, organic fruits and vegetables, have many beneficial phytochemicals. Tomatoes, for example, are thought to contain over

10,000 different phytochemicals. Fiber and numerous other benefits to be derived from eating whole foods (as opposed to *refined* foods) are the reason why whole foods are the way to go.

You will not experience the sugar slump with the whole grain bread that you will with the donut. The donut is like a hypodermic needle injecting sugar directly into your blood; the whole grain bread is more like a time-released capsule. It gives you the slow, sustained energy release you need. When the fuel in your system begins to wane, you will be signalled with hunger pangs that start slowly, instead of all of a sudden being so low on energy that you feel the urge to take a nap.

Unfortunately, many people, if they consume sugar like this regularly, end up in a constant up and down of energy, insulin, and glucose levels. This is hard on the body. When you feel that energy crash 60 to 90 minutes or so after consuming the donut, you may be inclined to reach for coffee or another donut, or anything you can get your hands on at a drive-through window or at the vending machine in the hallway. Understand that you cannot expect to be healthy or feel energetic this way, and that you are increasing your risk for numerous diseases. You will also likely carry extra weight.

Think of fiber in food as acting like a "brake" on the uptake of glucose into the blood. Another added benefit of fiber (and most of us don't get nearly enough) is that it will soak up and help the elimination of toxins and other undesirable food waste from the large intestine or colon. When these toxins are disposed of with fiber, they have less chance of working their way backwards from the large intestine into your small intestine. Your small intestine is where much of the absorption of food takes place. Okay, I have to back up again. Here's how the whole process of digestion begins.

When you chew food, your saliva secretes enzymes which begin the digestion process, particularly digestion of starches. After you swallow your (well-chewed!) food, the *peristaltic* action (kneading or massaging motion) of your *esophagus* pushes it down toward your stomach. At the bottom of your esophagus, where it meets your stomach, there is a sort of a valve, or flap of tissue, which prevents food from travelling back up towards your mouth. There are exceptions to this of course—when digestion goes wrong—but we'll talk about that later.

Once in your stomach, the powerful digestive enzymes and, in particular, hydrochloric acid, do the work of turning the food into what's called chyme. Little by little, chyme is released into your duodenum, the beginning of your small intestine, where the peristaltic action continues. Usable nutrients are absorbed here in the small intestine (which has a huge surface area and is very permeable). Indigestible fiber and foreign matter pass into the large intestine for removal. All the blood in your small intestine, mixed with the nutrients, toxins, fats, and other matter that were present in the food you just ate, now travels to the liver. The liver is like a big clean-up processing plant. Some of the many functions your liver cells perform:

- Neutralizes toxins;
- Makes bile salts;
- Deactivates hormones;
- Lowers or raises the sugar levels of your blood by responding to the commands of your pancreas;
- Oxidizes fats for energy;
- Produces cholesterol, phospholipids, and lipoproteins;
- Changes sugars and amino acids (protein) into fats;
- Uses vitamin K to make blood coagulation factors;
- Activates vitamin D.

These are just some of the many functions your liver performs. If it isn't functioning in top form, many health problems can result. These range from indigestion, bad breath, bloating, weight gain, low energy, or itchy skin—to the beginning stages of autoimmune diseases like diabetes, inflammatory bowel disease, and rheumatoid arthritis. It is impossible to overestimate or overstate the importance of liver health to the overall health and condition of your body.

When you become bloated after eating a large meal, this is a sign that your liver can't keep up with detoxification of the food you've just ingested. Remember, by "toxins," we don't mean literal poisons like arsenic or mercury (although we get traces of such toxins, as well). We are talking, partially at least, about the chemicals that are released in the breakdown of food. Some foods are much worse than others. For example, deep fryer fats, which are used repeatedly and recycled, are possibly the worst assault to your body. These fats have suffered extensive damage, to the point where they can be considered toxic (because they are repeatedly heated to high temperature and also kept at those high temperatures for long periods, perhaps days). Hard margarine is another *real* no-no. Both of these fats contain a type of fatty acid the body doesn't know how to respond to. This fat is *trans fat*, a substance completely foreign to the body. You know all about trans fats from the last chapter.

When these oils are in their pure form—liquid, unprocessed, organic, not subjected to heat or light, and, preferably, cold pressed—they are good for you (eaten in moderation). *Cold pressed* refers to the method by which the oil is extracted from the seed. This is not done by hexane extraction—a process which creates *free radicals*. (More on free radicals in Chapter 6.) When you make stir-fries for dinner (we're getting ahead of ourselves again, we were still on that donut you *weren't* having for breakfast), the canola or corn oil you use to fry up vegetables and chicken is oxidizing as it is heating. This oxidation is not good for you. You can limit the amount of damage heating an oil does by keeping the temperature of the oil below 212°F and by adding lots of garlic and onion to your meal. These two ingredients are high in *antioxidants* and will help counter-effect the oxidation taking place in the heated oil. Start by cooking everything in a little water and then add the oil later (for most stir-fries, a tablespoon or two should suffice).

Okay, back to your breakfast. Let's say you're like most people. You eat a couple of slices of toast, maybe a bit of yogurt, and then dash out the door. You're late, so you're stressed. This stress constricts your blood vessels, promoting high blood pressure, and makes your breathing more shallow, which causes a whole host of problems. When you neglect to breathe deeply, your diaphragm does not fully engage, which means it does not act upon the liver and your other digestive organs, massaging them and stimulating them to work in top form. You do not get the oxygen you should be getting, which means your cells are being deprived of their most vital nutrient. If you smoke, all this is intensified many times over.

As you are driving, feeling frustrated at the traffic jams and seeming to catch all the red lights, your stomach, small intestine, pancreas, liver, and gallbladder are working hard to digest your toast and yogurt. As already mentioned, all the blood that leaves your small intestine goes first through the liver before moving to the heart and brain. Therefore, you can see the problems that develop if you overtax your liver! The liver has what might be called "inlet" and "outlet" valves which control the flow of blood … you guessed it … into and out of the liver. When you feel bloated after a meal, your liver inlet valves have shut down because your liver is running behind on its detoxification process. It usually doesn't take long for the liver to catch up—when it does, the inlet valves open up and things quickly return to normal. Of course, certain enzymes and other crucial substances, like vitamins and hormones, must exist for the liver to function in top form.

Your outlet valves shut down for the same reason. Your immune system is set up in such a way as to ensure that your liver is essentially your first line of defense. However, it has its limits. In cases of severe liver damage, such as with cirrhosis or

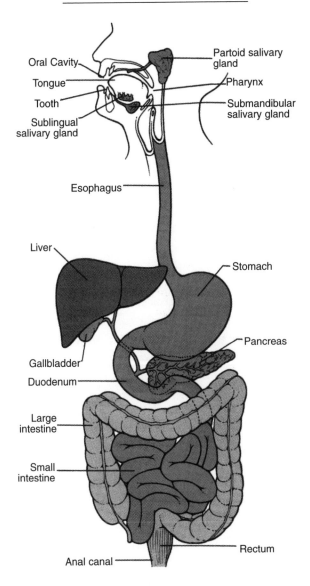

Your Digestive System: Notice the many salivary glands that play a role in the digestion of your food. If you don't chew your foods properly, you are forcing your stomach to do more digestive work than it was designed to do. Indigestion is often the result.

hepatitis, we see the liver retaining fluid—the mixture of bile salts, toxins, fats, proteins, and so on—to the point where the liver becomes enlarged. If the liver still cannot keep up by "bloating up" while detoxification catches up, toxins end up in your bloodstream. When you have an excess mucous condition, such as when you have a cold, it is—indirectly at least—your body's response to an overtaxed liver.

Every drop of your blood filters through your liver every four minutes, so you can see how efficient the liver has to be! When the liver can no longer cope with the flood of toxins, and the liver outlet valves are shut as a result, the liver has no choice but to dump these fluids directly into your bile or into your sinusoids—the spaces around the detoxifying liver cells. This toxic bile, which is overburdening the liver, will now be dumped into your immune system, then concentrated in your gallbladder, which over time becomes very irritated. Your gallbladder is stimulated to release bile to the duodenum to aid in digestion—particularly of fats—after a meal. When this bile is toxic, it not only irritates the gallbladder but also weakens the membranes in your duodenum. These membranes then become more susceptible to attack from the bacteria in your colon. We have billions of bacteria in the colon which are absolutely vital to good health. However, some of this bacteria is not of a nature you'd want sneaking backwards through your digestive system. It should stay in the colon in preparation for removal with your next bowel movement. This is why fiber is so important—you want to get rid of this bacteria *as quickly as possible*. Fiber also feeds friendly (or beneficial) bacteria, which makes vitamin B12, detoxifies, and in turn feeds on fiber containing useful by-products.

Some people, when they have indigestion or heartburn after a meal, reach for antacids. The theory is that the stomach is making too much acid and must be "calmed down." While your stomach *may* be making too much acid, it is probably more likely the case that the toxic bile, normally stored in the gallbladder (setting the stage for gall stones), is irritating your duodenum so much, that acid is leaking out of your stomach and travelling up your esophagus. The answer is to clean up the liver and by extension the gallbladder, and then to eat healthy, whole food.

By the way, if you are reading this hoping to hear that there is a safe way to eat lots of donuts and bacon, you'll be disappointed. If you truly want to be healthy, feel younger, be more energetic, and live longer, there are certain no-option rules. But we guarantee the trip is well worth it, and the "sacrifices" you will make will not even feel like sacrifices once you are on the road to good health. Stay with us. We'll take you there.

Now, where were we? Oh, yes. You're driving to work. You arrive with a few minutes to spare and your first stop is the lunchroom to see if anyone's put on a pot of coffee. Someone has. Bless their soul. You pour a cup and head to your desk. Now, let's see. What do you do for a living? Where do you live? This offers an opportunity to illustrate what you might eat and drink, and how you might organize your day differently, may depend on the type of work you do, and on where you live.

Some experts recommend starting your day with fruit, and eating nothing but fruit until noon. While we believe firmly in the benefits of fruit and in particular starting your day with it (remember: fluids, fiber, food energy, and vitamin C—an apple or orange would provide all four), the body needs more than fruit to kick-start the day. Considerations:

(a) Fruit is high in fructose (a type of sugar) and some bodies cannot handle the sugar well enough without the counterbalancing effects of either starch, fiber, or protein. Your best breakfast will provide a combination of carbohydrates, proteins, and fats. Some suggestions:
- Carbohydrates (whole grain cereal or toast—though many of today's health complaints stem from allergies to *wheat*—more on allergies in Chapter 3);

- *Fresh* fruit;
- Some type of hot cereal like slow-cooked rolled oats (not the instant kind which is just mush and has had all its beneficial fiber and nutrients stripped, then added back in);
- Cold, high-fiber cereal like bran flakes, or muesli you make yourself, with 2% cow's, goat's or soy milk;
- A bowl of brown rice sprinkled with raisins and nuts;
- One or two hard-boiled or poached (not fried) *free-range eggs*, chewed well. Eggs provide fat and protein;
- Cheese—from a variety of sources: cow's milk, goat's milk, and soy. Cheese also provides protein and fat;
- If you must spread something onto your bread, try:
  - peanut butter or other nut butters;
  - mashed avocado mixed with green onions, a little fresh lemon juice, and freshly ground pepper;
  - stewed fresh fruit with a small amount of raw, unpasteurized honey;
  - real maple syrup, for those of you with a sweet tooth (do *not* eat sugary, commercially prepared jams and jellies);
- A small amount of butter is acceptable, unless you are liver cleansing, in which case you want to avoid not only all dairy products, but certainly your diet should be 90-95% free of saturated fats for the duration of your cleansing program. Hard margarine should never be consumed. There are a few margarines, such as Becel®, which provide beneficial poly-unsaturated fats and are not hydrogenated. Choose such margarines over others.

(b) If you live in a northern climate, you would probably be wise to take a supplement of vitamin D in the winter. A deficiency in vitamin D can also lead to a deficiency in calcium, as vitamin D is needed for the retention of calcium. (By the way, that cup of coffee you're having at your desk right now will also rob your body of calcium). Another important note: please do not use coffee whiteners. They are not made from milk; they are made from hydrogenated vegetable oils and are very high in trans fats.

(c) If you have a physically demanding job, eat accordingly. Again, the key is common sense. Carbohydrates will supply your body with the required energy to get you through the morning and will also give your brain the fuel it needs if you have a mentally demanding job. However, protein consumed with carbohydrates will give longer-lasting energy, and this energy will also be more available for use by the muscles, if you have a physical sort of job. This is also the reason why you should consume *something* before you work out in the morning. Vitamin C is best taken before a workout because of its antioxidant properties.

(d) If you struggle with weight, we'll try to correct that in the chapter on liver cleansing. In the meantime, your breakfast should be a mix of approximately 40% carbohydrates, 30% protein, and 30% fat (most of your diet should follow this ratio). You can alter the percentage of fat to 20% and increase the carbohydrates and/or protein by 10% if you are trying to shed unwanted pounds. If all this sounds like you will be weighing every crumb of food, rest assured, we will not ask you to resort to measuring portions or counting fat grams or calories. You *will* need to be aware of how much you're consuming every day, because it's important to "measure" how much fat you're eating, but once you understand the easy eating program, this will become second nature to you.

The fat you eat at *any* of your meals, but probably most importantly at breakfast, should be high in essential fatty acids. You know all about essential fatty acids already. Foods high in EFAs are flax seed and flax seed oil, fish, dark, leafy green vegetables, nuts, and whole grains.

Let's assume you have a desk job, because most of us suffer from lifestyles that are too sedentary anyway. You are in a job where many of the decisions are not yours to make, yet you bear a lot of responsibility, and this adds to your stress. We'll also assume that you are slightly overweight, and slightly out of shape. You can be either male or female—most of the principles put forward in this book will apply more or less equally to both genders. You are in your early 30's to mid-50's, and you live in the city. Studies have shown that married people are healthier, on average, than single people (particularly men). However, for the purposes of our discussions, you can either be married or not, and you may or may not have children.

We're attempting to draw a picture of a typical person who might be in need of a health boost. If you are a 20-year old college student, a pensioner who lives alone, 30-ish, 40-ish, or 50-ish but you have never been married and you don't intend to ever have children, these principles still apply. Whether you work construction, are a dentist, a child care worker, a philosopher, a gourmet coffee clerk—of any age—these principles will apply to you as well. Where you must use caution and check with your doctor, and where generalizations we will have to make may not apply at all, is if you are suffering from a degenerative disease like diabetes, cancer, arthritis, heart disease, kidney disease, or multiple sclerosis. You should also bear in mind that if you make changes to your diet and level of activity, do so *slowly and gradually*. Another concept we will try to make clear to you is that of *balance*. Nothing of any lasting greatness can be achieved if you overdo it in any area of life. You can even eat too many vegetables, and it is easy to overdo exercise, especially if you have been sedentary for some time.

Okay, back to the task at hand, which is discussing digestion in the average person, on an average day, for a person with an average sort of job and life. Hopefully all this "average-ness" doesn't sound dull, but most of you wouldn't be able to relate to a discussion about the health of a long-distance marathon runner or a 10-year old growing up in the country.

You are at your desk and you finished your coffee (which was ice cold) about 20 minutes ago. You're reasonably moderate so you don't immediately go for another cup the way many would. Your adrenal gland has just flooded your system with adrenalin and you are feeling the rush now. You figure you'll make it through until noon. It's 10:30. You work for an insurance firm and you are regularly required to deal with the public. They visit you to discuss their insurance needs. Many people you see have obvious health problems: they are severely overweight, or are too thin; they are smokers and are wheezing from the walk down the hall; the older ladies are stooped from osteoporosis; some people your age (late 30's) yawn through the whole session; when you shake their hands you notice their skin is clammy or scaly and dry; they have bad breath; circles under their eyes; dull hair; a pale, drawn look to their skin and eyes. You have started asking questions about your own health: you read articles on health in the popular literature, wondering whether your diet will protect you from osteoporosis, fearing menopause and all its attendant problems (if you're a woman). If you're male, you've worried about prostate cancer or maybe that spare tire around your waist.

In an aging society, we must learn to take more responsibility for our own health. We simply cannot do all the things we'd like to do because they "feel good"—smoking, drinking (too much alcohol or coffee), or regularly eating fatty desserts. Other health-robbing habits many of us fall into we feel we cannot avoid. They are a "necessary evil". These "fact of life" issues may be due to overcommitment on our part—depriving ourselves of sleep and rest, and avoiding exercise are the results. Many of us fall victim to all the syndromes: we don't sleep enough or get enough rest. We are so busy we do not have time to cook healthful meals, and we compensate for our lack of energy and ability to concentrate with cigarettes and coffee.

We cannot expect to be healthy with so much working against us. And we cannot expect to have all these bad habits and then, when illness strikes, expect a doctor or bottle of pills to make us well again. No vitamin, mineral, or other health food supplement; no drug, taken in pill powder, lotion or potion form, holds the key to good health, to being lean and fit, to renewed youth and vigor.

Vibrant health and longevity depend on a *whole-body* approach. A *lifestyle* approach. A *lifelong* approach. And there is *no way* around this. Again, sorry if this disappoints you, but you will see that the "sacrifices" are *so* worth the rewards. You won't be sorry.

It is 11:00. Your body has assimilated the nutrients you gave it at breakfast, now four hours ago. If you are trying to lose weight, the general rule is that if you have had a large meal in the last four hours, you don't need to eat. But hard and fast rules aren't good. You should instead learn to listen to your body's cues. This can take some practice to do well. Most of us are flooded with cues from other sources: the media, boredom, stress. You should eat only if you are hungry, and stop when you are full.

Now, at mid-morning and at least an hour before lunch, are you hungry? Then eat something. But come prepared. Instead of heading into the hallway or to the corner store to buy sugary or salty junk food, bring fruit or mixed raw nuts from home. Or cut up vegetables. Most grocery stores now sell washed, cut, and trimmed vegetables, ready for consumption. They're a little more expensive than the other kind (the kind that require work), but it might be worth it if it's the only way you'll eat your veggies.

In order to protect against cancer, you should be eating a variety of at least five to ten servings of richly-colored fruits and vegetables every day. Your best bets: citrus fruits and beta-carotene-rich foods such as orange/yellow/dark green vegetables and the cruciferous (cabbage) vegetables. These all have the added benefit of being high in fiber.

You've brought an apple for your morning snack? Excellent. Eat it slowly. Don't swallow a lot of air. Chew it well. Apples are an excellent source of potassium, and a fair source of vitamin C. Now your metabolism can rev up again—it has something to do! Now it can burn calories again because your internal heat generator has been activated! Does that make sense? That's why you want to keep your metabolism working at a high rate.

Speaking of metabolism, consider this. You've heard people at the gym say that it's important when you're starting a workout regimen to include weight training, especially if you're a woman. This is true. After the age of 35, women lose a pound of muscle every year unless they consciously build muscle to counteract that.

When the body is at rest, muscles burn far more calories than fat because they are more metabolically active. Muscle also weighs more than fat. If you start on a fitness routine and you are weight training along with cardiovascular exercise to burn fat, *weight loss* may appear to go slowly. You have lost *fat*, but gained *muscle*. A better indicator of your success is how many inches you've lost or simply how well your jeans fit. Also, many gyms and fitness centres have machines that quickly and easily calculate the amount of fat and lean tissue in your body.

Let's say you've determined you need to lose weight and you started out at 40 pounds over your ideal weight. You power walk several hours every week, you swim, and you weight train for about 45 minutes two to three times a week. While the cardio-vascular exercise you are doing will certainly mean you will lose fat, the strength training you are doing also means you are gaining muscle. Since muscle weighs more than fat, you may see the numbers on the scale drop more slowly than you feel they should be dropping. A good rule of thumb: *stay off the scale.* Do not focus on numbers. What constitutes the right weight for someone else doesn't necessarily constitute the right weight for you.

Now, a few more words about muscle. A body that has a high percentage of muscle burns fuel more efficiently and more quickly (read: you can eat more and not gain weight). Muscle will help reduce your risk of injury—for instance, lifting a heavy box, hauling your 2-year old up onto your hip a hundred times a day, or scrubbing out your bathtub. With good muscle tone, you are far less likely to pull something, pinch a nerve, or lose your balance and fall. When you are older, this muscle power will help keep you from breaking bones and will help keep your posture upright.

Now, you've made it to lunch. And, horrors! You feel you are too busy to step away from your desk to regenerate, and so you work through until your hunger pangs subside. You don't do this often, but a pile of work has just landed on your desk, and you have to leave early today because you have to pick up your son from school to take him to a doctor's appointment. Now, here's what's going on inside your body.

Your metabolism started slowing down as soon as that apple was digested. Fruit only takes about 20 minutes to work its way through your system; nothing is digested more quickly when eaten on an empty stomach. Your pancreas has detected low levels of glucose in your blood, so it sends a message to your liver via the hormone *glucagon* to release sugars stored there. You also store glucose in your muscles, but this is usually only released when you are really taxing your body, like when you are out jogging. The picture looks like this: if you are a woman with a reasonably sedentary lifestyle, your calorie requirement is under 2,000 calories per day. Right now, because you have skipped lunch, you are forcing your body to run on about 400 calories, given what you've eaten (remember: toast and yogurt for breakfast, an apple at about 11:00). While the glucose released from your liver will keep you functioning, it will not keep you functioning in top form. You will feel tired, you brain will feel sluggish, you will not be able to think clearly, and you will be very short on energy. This may prompt you to reach for another cup of coffee.

Okay, now you'll feel better for a little while. It's 2:30 and you have to leave to pick up your son from school. You have a slight headache (low blood sugar) and your stomach feels off

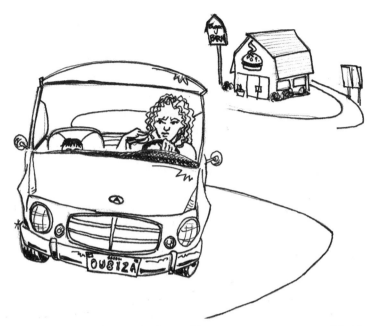

(you have irritated it with the coffee on an empty stomach). You pick up your son, but he doesn't have to be to his appointment until 3:30. You're both hungry, so you stop at a fast food burger drive-through on your way.

You are now going to hit your body with about 1,300 calories. So many people kid themselves when they buy fast food, too. They order the big behemoth burger, french fries, and then a diet pop. Some sandwich places aren't much better. One fast food sandwich shop makes a tuna sub that has 56 grams of fat! To put this into perspective, a lean cut of beef can have as little as 4 grams of fat, a glass of 2% milk has just 5. Moreover, if you are consuming about 1,800 calories per day for weight maintenance, you can easily put yourself over with just one meal consumed at the Burger Barn.

Let's stop here a moment and look more closely at calories. We have fixated over the last 20 years on how much fat we consume and so we have cut fat out of our diets. Here's what's wrong with this picture. We've all heard it: fat makes you fat. Well, so do carbohydrates. The difference between fat and carbohydrates is that fat must first be stored in the body before it can be used, whereas carbohydrates are used directly and immediately. BUT, if you consume more calories in the form of carbohydrates than your body requires, they are converted into glucose for storage in the liver and in the muscles. If there are simply too many sugars, your body will convert the rest into fatty acids, which are then packaged into triglycerides and sent off via the blood to the fat tissues for storage. So, along with fat, you must be aware of the carbohydrates you consume as well. Too much protein can also cause problems (especially in the absence of carbohydrates).

If you are trying to lose weight, your fat consumption should be in the neighborhood of 20 to 25 per cent of your caloric intake per day. You may think it better to get away with less, like about 15 to 20 per cent, but it is difficult to feel satisfied with fat intakes below 20% of total energy intake. If you are maintaining your present weight, your fat consumption should be in the 30 per cent range. Remember, the quality of the fat you consume is more important than the quantity you consume. Saturated fatty acids are found primarily in animal products such as dairy items, beef, veal, lamb, and pork. Some vegetable oils—coconut, palm kernel, and vegetable shortening—are also high in saturates.[2] You should limit your consumption of this type of fat to well under 10 per cent per day. In Chapter 1, you learned all about which types of fats are good for you and why.

Polyunsaturated fatty acids are found in corn, soybean, safflower, and sunflower oils. These fats have a tendency to lower overall blood cholesterol, but in doing so also lower your HDLs (high density lipoproteins), which are vital to your good health. These fats, too, should not constitute more than 10 per cent of your total caloric intake. Don't believe everything you read about cholesterol, however. You do need it for good health.

Monounsaturated fatty acids are found mostly in nuts, olives, peanuts (and their oils) and in canola oil. These appear to lower LDL (low density lipoproteins) cholesterol as well, but have no effect on HDL cholesterol. However, even with this apparent good news, all fats are high in calories (9 per gram) and so should be factored into the daily percentage, good or bad.

Trans fats are much harder to figure out from labels (you have to do some arithmetic). If you look at a label for mayonnaise, for example, you will see a total energy measure per serving. I'll use a brand we all know well. It has 65 calories per serving. A serving is one tablespoon. The table below shows how to do the math:

Serving Size: 1 Tablespoon, Total Calories per Serving: 65

Protein	0.1 g
Fat	6.5 g*
Polyunsaturates	1.9 g
Monounsaturates	3.8 g
Saturates	0.5 g
Cholesterol	7 mg

*Total calories from fat—at 9 calories per gram—per serving: 58.5 calories or 90% calories from fat

---

The cholesterol in this product is negligible. Three types of fats add up to 6.2 grams. However, total fat is 6.5 grams. If you subtract those 6.2 grams of fat from the total fat (6.5 grams), you get the amount of trans fat in the product, in this case .3 grams. Now, as mayonnaise goes, this is not bad. It is very low in cholesterol and very low in trans fats. Trans fats are the worst type of fat you can consume. That's why you should stay away from all hard margarines and products like many salad dressings, instant puddings, muffin and cake mixes, and a whole host of other packaged foods (including some that seem healthy, like boxed granola) because of their high *hydrogenated vegetable oil* or *partially hydrogenated vegetable oil* content. This is what you should look for on a label. Stay away from these foods.

The method to arrive at the percentage trans fats can also illustrate how to arrive at the percentage of calories from fat in the product. Simply take the total fat grams, multiply by 9 (all fats contain 9 calories per gram) and divide this number by the total number of calories per serving. In the case of the mayonnaise example, you would divide the total number of calories from fat (58.5) by the total number of calories in the serving (65) to arrive at .9 or 90%. Of course, it's no surprise that mayonnaise is 90% fat, but do this math with some of the common products you have around your house, and you'll be shocked at the fat content of many foods. And when you select products at the grocery store, don't be fooled by "lite" or "low fat" labels—they can be very misleading. Remember the percentage fat intake range you want to stay within for your level of activity (as we discussed earlier). This is relatively easy to do with packaged foods that have this information listed on the label, but it can't help you when you are buying fast food items or bakery products. The solution: stay away from these foods.

When you understand how the math works, you then have the ammunition when you are negotiating with your spouse about whether or not you will even *buy* that salad dressing, or which type to buy, and it will arm you with much needed information when your kids are begging for the latest breakfast cereal. However, we've promised you that you won't need to do any math, and we'll stick by that promise. But knowledge is power. Tuck that little fat/calorie/trans fat figuring system into your subconscious.

Now, let's look back for a moment to the trip to the Burger Barn. You've blown your caloric count for the day—*big time*. Worse, you've eaten very quickly (remember, you're in your car on the way to your son's doctor's appointment). Now, let's see what we've done with our allowable fat count for the day. A bacon cheeseburger contains about 40 grams of fat—almost half of which are saturated[3]. A regular order of fries will run about 12 grams of fat, about 4 grams of which are saturated. The burger has 609 calories, the fries 235. A chocolate milkshake rounds out your (lunch? dinner?) with 320 more calories to add to the list. That's 1,254 calories, 44 per cent of which are from fat.

If you have any digestive upset problems at all, like a low functioning gallbladder, gastroesophageal reflux disease, irritable bowel, or you simply suffer from the myriad of low-grade chronic health problems collectively known as "indigestion," you will really suffer from a meal like this. Here's why.

Digestion should happen thoroughly. This is very important. Have you ever had a heavy, fatty, or extraordinarily spicy meal, which you are still burping up hours later? Everything you eat has to be converted to a form usable by the body. The liver plays a large role in this. So, when you eat a meal like the one from the Burger Barn, you will make the liver work hard no matter how healthy you are.

After all the food has been ingested, it makes its way to the small intestine. Once there, every drop of blood—carrying toxins, nutrients, and partly digested proteins—passes through your portal vein to be processed by your liver. The more toxins (or damaged fats) you put into your body at once, the harder your liver has to work. Hard-to-digest fats, in particular, will wreak havoc with your liver, especially if your liver enzymes are not working in top form.

By the way, if you feel that your liver is not working in top form, you may want to have your blood tested for liver enzymes. This is best done with a naturopathic physician, since the tests that orthodox medicine conduct are sometimes too crude to establish subtle (but important) problems with liver function.

This meal is the worst kind of assault to your liver. Most fast food places now use vegetable shortening; some use beef lard. This fat is kept at high heats for very, very long periods of time and so is damaged to a great degree. It is also recycled—the extent of the damage done to this fat can't even be imagined. Ironically, beef tallow is better for you when used for deep-frying, than vegetable oils. Tallow, even when heated and recycled, will not change its molecular structure the way vegetable oil will. Either way, though, deep-frying is a terrible way to cook food.

Deep-frying food soaks what was once a humble, nutritious item (such as the potato) into fattening, toxic, non-nutritious junk. The fat in the meat and the dressings or sauces used in the burger (including the *processed* cheese) are either saturated fat or trans fats, neither of which will do your body any favours, though the trans fats are always worse. Because this meal is very low in fiber, any of the toxins and indigestible matter that has now passed into your large intestine for disposal, might sit there for awhile without any bulk to move it out. The milkshake you had contains lots of sugar. In the small intestine, it is converted to glucose and either used for energy or sent off to the fat deposit centers of your body. If the Burger Barn uses real milk to make their milkshakes (no guarantee of that, though), this may be the most nutrition you are getting from this "meal". The sugar and white flour feed the bad bacteria in your bowel, unless you have a good balance of beneficial intestinal flora (good bacteria), that inhibits bacterial overgrowth.

After your appointment, you are still burping up what tastes like a combination of bile and french fries. Actually, that's exactly what it is. When you eat fats, your gallbladder is stimulated to release bile to aid in their digestion. Bile makes fats more water soluble so that enzymes can do their job. Bile salts and lecithin are the key ingredients that weaken the fat globules so that the kneading action of your intestine can make smaller particles out of them. Bile salts can be sent directly to your duodenum from your liver or they can be stored in your gallbladder.

In order for your gallbladder to store bile it must concentrate it—that is, it must remove most of the water from it first. If you have toxic bile due to an overloaded liver that is dumping toxins out into your bile because it can't keep up, your gallbladder and entire digestive system will become aggravated every time you eat, but especially when you eat a fatty meal.

The good news is that with a proper diet, you can reverse much of this damage. You can dissolve gallstones (this is not guaranteed, but certainly possible), clean up your liver, regenerate liver cells, and return your body to a state of health. Even if you decide you are going to have your gallbladder or gallstones surgically removed (which is sometimes necessary), there is no guarantee that fats will never bother you in the future. Symptoms may return after surgery, if you continue to eat the same way.

There are other vital components to digestion, of course. Good circulation, enzymes, vitamins, minerals, water, and movement are all essential to *proper and complete* digestion of food. If you follow the eating plan laid out for you in Chapter 4, you stand a reasonable chance of getting most of the nutrients you need from your food. However, we advocate supplementation as it is virtually impossible for people living in today's world to eat according to this plan one hundred per cent of the time. The vitamins, minerals, and enzymes you need are outlined in Chapter 6. There is a very effective way to ensure your stomach has enough hydrochloric acid to handle digestion of food. Each morning, on an empty stomach, take two tablespoons of apple cider vinegar (the kind from the health food store) in a half glass of tepid water. This will restore the acid balance in your system.

Now, where were we? Your son's appointment has revealed unpleasant, though not terrible, news about allergies he appears to have. You bundle him back into the car and by now you are sniffling and you have sneezed several times. You curse your high heels as you splash through a puddle at the foot of the driver's door of your car. As you drive home, you consider how you will handle the allergies your son has. You could have further testing done, but how much would that cost, and where would you go? How will it affect what you cook at home, what you pack for his lunch?

In Chapter 3, we will discuss allergies in some detail so that you will not only understand them but also have an idea of what you can do about them.

You arrive home—a little earlier than usual—and collapse onto the couch. You've got 20 minutes before your daughter arrives home from daycare. Your husband won't be home for over an hour. You've been worried about him lately. You've heard so much about prostate health, and he's carrying a little bit of extra weight as well. High blood pressure runs in his family and you've tried—and failed—to convince him to give up mayonnaise on his sandwiches, chips, and beer with his ball games.

The truth is, a little mayonnaise, chips, or beer isn't going to kill anyone. Though we don't advocate eating these foods on a regular basis, if you are in reasonably good health, they certainly aren't going to have a huge adverse effect on your health either. Again, we must revisit the concept of balance. You can, paradoxically, make things worse for yourself if you worry too much about what you are eating, when, in what quantities, and whether these foods will make you sick, fat, or diseased. Enjoy a beer once in a while. Have ice cream if you are enjoying a day at the fairgrounds with your family. But *enjoy* these foods when you have them. Don't become so consumed with guilt that you don't enjoy the food anymore. What's the point in that? If you can't eat it guilt-free, then don't eat it. And if you are the type of person that isn't even tempted, better yet. Pack a bowl of fruit salad and sandwiches made with lots of veggies to the fairgrounds and have a picnic lunch instead. The point is … don't fret over every little thing. If you have a "bad" food once in a while, it's okay. This is especially true if you are eating out with friends. Everybody is sharing several different plates of finger food, but you pick at a salad because of how "bad" you know all that food is. This isn't fun, and it's not living.

We don't want to create a picture of abstinence that you may be seeing with all these foods you allegedly are not allowed to eat. You're probably screaming, *So many foods have bad fats, is there anything left to eat that's fun?* The answer is … yes. And no.

If you are ill now, you must first take steps to correct your illness before you worry about whether food can ever be fun again. If you have digestive upset now because of an irritated gallbladder or sluggish liver, you may have to forgo "fun" foods completely for a few months while you give your body a chance to heal. If you've ever had a gallbladder attack, though—especially after a seemingly innocuous meal—fun food wouldn't be of as much concern to you. If you're severely overweight and your doctor has told you that you are at high risk for gallstones, diabetes, heart disease, or certain forms of cancer, you ought not to be worried at all about having fun with food. Instead you should heal your body first. You *will* have fun again. Most of you will be allowed to eat those certain foods, on occasion at least, that bring so much pleasure—chocolate, wine, potato chips, cookies, ice cream. So don't worry, stay with us.

You have decided to make a salad for dinner. Great! You pick iceberg lettuce, tomatoes, carrots, and radishes. You sprinkle on grated cheddar and then get out the bottled dressings—there's Thousand Islands, French, Buttermilk, and a raspberry vinaigrette that looks deceptively low fat. You choose the raspberry vinaigrette; your son, whom you suspect is allergic to wheat, takes the Thousand Islands, your daughter hates salad dressings and instead picks tomato slices and carrots out of the bowl.

Unfortunately, your salad is only moderately nutritious. You score points for choosing salad in the first place, and perhaps also for the type of dressing (is it low fat? what type of fat does it contain?) but you could do better by altering those choices slightly.

When making salad, try to use spinach, green leaf, or romaine lettuce. Iceberg lettuce, while containing some nutrition, is a poorer choice. Your son is eating Thousand Islands dressing. Did you know that many of these types of products contain wheat designed to thicken them? Later, when he gets stuffed up and sleepy you'll wonder why—after all, he didn't eat any bread at all today, so far as you know (you're already forgotten about that hamburger, haven't you?).

When your husband arrives home, he heats leftovers. You made a chicken stir-fry last night and there's just enough for him. You had decided to save it for him. The kids aren't happy with just salad so you make them each a grilled cheese sandwich, forgetting, again, (it's okay, you're only human) your son's wheat allergy, and the fact that cheese seems to give your daughter nightmares. You yourself are still too full from the hamburger and in fact have had a slightly upset stomach ever since. Your sniffling has gotten worse and you are now stuffed up. You've heard that echinacea is good for the onset of a cold, but you don't have any in the house. You have some vitamin C and E, but you haven't taken either in weeks. You consider staying home the next day, but then realize you can't because you have an important lunch meeting.

You have probably been fighting this cold for close to a week. Because your diet is below optimal, your body is constantly deprived of the nutrients it needs for many different functions—immune support, proper digestion, and assimilation of the nutrients you do get. Your schedule of six hours sleep a night is not enough for the body to go about its repair work and to create the hormones you need to be alert and awake the next day. Your habit of too much coffee dehydrates you and depletes your body of many important minerals, setting the stage for conditions such as osteoporosis to develop later in life. If you're a woman, coffee makes PMS and menstrual cramps worse.

Dehydration, another condition coffee worsens, is a serious

problem many people do not give enough thought to. The body is about 70% water. All the important functions of digestion, absorption, excretion of waste, and other metabolic processes, such as cell division and manufacture, happen in a watery medium. When you are dehydrated, you force these functions to take place in a sub-optimal environment. The result is … sub-optimal results. When you don't consume enough water (and no, coffee and black tea do not count as water), your body retains the water it has. What this means is that any of the toxins (including cold and flu bacteria and viruses) and old cells that are circulating in your body will not be eliminated as quickly. But do not confuse this. When you drink a lot of coffee and you have to go to pee a lot, this is not the same as drinking lots of water and having to pee a lot. Coffee, when expelled, carries with it important minerals, as we've said. You may get fluids when you drink coffee and tea, but the caffeine counteracts any good the fluid is doing. Even decaffeinated coffee has taken hits lately and is not without negative effects. The same goes for caffeinated colas. Here you get a double hit: caffeine *and* sugar. If you think you are doing yourself a favour with diet pop, think again. No one knows for sure whether aspartame is safe (in some reports it has been shown to cause an increase in brain tumours), and in any event it is a substance your liver will struggle with, a substance it must neutralize and detoxify. The best thing in pop is the water and, again, the substances in the pop you don't want will nullify the benefits you might get from the fluid. Do yourself a favour—save the money and drink water.

You want whatever goes in to go out pretty quickly (not the way it does with laxatives: that is unnaturally quick and does not give your body time to absorb the nutrients). But you do want digestion and absorption to work quickly. First of all, your metabolism will stay running at a high rate, nutrients will be absorbed quickly, and you will feel full faster when you eat, helping you to control your weight. Waste matter, which is toxic—we all know that now, right?—will be excreted from the body quickly. Remember, if toxins sit in your colon without bulk to move them out, eventually those toxins are either absorbed through the walls of the colon and into your bloodstream or they will travel backwards into your small intestine, where your liver is forced to work them over again. Then, if your liver becomes overtaxed with its detoxification work, it in effect throws up its hands and sends the toxins into your blood (this ends up in your sinuses, lymph, and bloodstream, wreaking havoc on tissues throughout your body).

In the same way a diet low in fiber will cause toxins to sit dangerously long in your colon, a diet low in water will cause toxins to sit dangerously long in your bladder. This can also cause health problems, particularly in men who are now seeing a rise in the incidence of prostate cancer.

Your kidneys do an admirable job filtering the liquid waste your body creates. If overtaxed, however, they respond the same way your liver does: but they simply dump toxins out through your skin. The result is body odor, rashes, acne, dandruff, dry, scaly skin, eczema, and general itching.

You should be drinking 8 to 12 glasses of water a day. The best water, in my opinion, is reverse osmosis (RO), but distilled is equally good from a health point of view. We just find that RO water tastes the best. Be careful with spring and tap water. Hard well water is acceptable in moderate quantities, and has recently been shown to be protective against heart disease. Hard tap water may be different, as you don't know the content or level of the minerals in it. The hardness scale of water refers to its mineral content—the harder it is, the more minerals it contains. While the body needs minerals in minute quantities to function, most of the minerals contained in well water are common and you are unlikely to ever suffer a deficiency of them. Minerals present in tap water can build up in body tissues and promote conditions like chronic fatigue syndrome and fibromyalgia. They can even

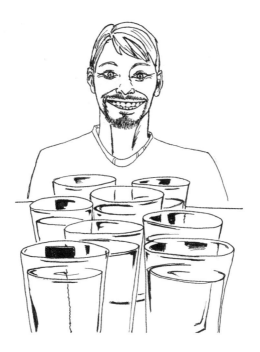

result in calcium deposits which can become inflamed and can be very painful. City or "treated" tap water usually also contains chlorine as an antibacterial agent to kill off bacteria like E. coli. You are lucky if you live in an area where water is purified through a process known as ozone treatment.

Tap water is fine in moderation, but, again, if you are on city-treated water, the level of chemicals you are consuming is unacceptable by most standards. You should know what's in your water—whether you are on a well or a city-treated system. Take a sample and have it tested.

Of course, the authorities will assure you everything is fine with your water. However, even though much of what can harm you has been killed off with chlorine, you are now faced with ingesting chlorine (yuck!). If you are in an area that gets high rainfall, you will often have turbid or cloudy water. You would avoid this water if you were hiking and bent at a stream to drink, so why would you consider it okay coming from your tap?

Buy a water cooler and stand it in the corner of your kitchen, and buy reverse osmosis or steam-distilled water for it. You will always have ice cold water at your fingertips and you know it will be pure and healthy.

On that note, there are a few appliances the health-conscious person shouldn't be without. One is a water cooler. Another is a juicer. Juicing is one of the best ways to get super-concentrated nutrition into your diet. It is also a must when you follow the liver cleansing program outlined in Chapter 4. Food processors are handy because when you eat a lot of fresh foods and prepare things yourself, they make life a whole lot simpler. A "house" in which to make sprouts is handy, though sprouting seeds is easy enough to do with a jar and some cheesecloth.

You wrap up your evening by reading the newspaper and watching TV. Your husband seems fine physically, but his job is really stressing him, and he hasn't found a way to control this, and he hasn't seen a doctor about it yet. You've heard that certain herbs can be good to control stress. What you both need to know is that without exercise, the right attitude (commitment and consistency), and clean, whole food, complete health—mental and physical—will never be possible. You must do the work to achieve good health. There are no shortcuts.

You retire after 11:00, knowing you will be tired the next day (you're up at 6:00). You already recognize the signs of being unable to fall asleep—your mind is distracted and churning with worries. Well after 12:30 you are still sniffling and you know that by morning you will have a full-blown cold. The lack of exercise in your life makes it harder to fall asleep at night. Tips for a good night's sleep:

- Use your bed only for sleep and sex;
- Go to bed at the same time every night and get up at the same time every morning. If you burn the midnight oil on the weekends and then sleep in the next day, on Monday you

will feel like you are getting up in the middle of the night;

- Don't try hard to fall asleep. Instead, languish and feel lazy;
- If you have trouble falling asleep, get up and do something—make a list, listen to quiet music, do some yoga, have a warm bath;
- Don't exercise in the two hours leading up to your bedtime;
- Don't eat anything for three to four hours before bedtime;
- Darken your room and quiet your surroundings. Try earplugs if there is noise from your neighbourhood or if your partner snores;
- Sleep in a well-ventilated room and don't pile on the blankets to the point where you are too warm;
- While you should drink 8-12 glasses of water daily, try not to drink much after 6:00 or 7:00 pm. You will have to get up to go to the bathroom too often;
- Don't drink any caffeinated drinks after about 3:00 or 4:00 in the afternoon;
- Avoid heavy foods at dinner or at any time before bed: foods high in fat—especially cheese and ice cream—will wreak havoc with your digestive system, keeping you awake and causing nightmares;
- If you really have trouble sleeping, try meditation (not *medication*) as part of your daily routine. It will teach you ways to quiet your mind;
- There are lots of herbs you can take that can help you sleep. Among them: kava kava, St. John's Wort, valerian, chamomile, spearmint, hops, passion flower. Calcium is said to be "nature's tranquilizer." Since supplementing with calcium is a good idea anyway, get some for yourself and take it with vitamin D, about an hour before going to bed.

Remember that good digestion—and by extension good health—starts and ends with common sense. Eat good foods, chew them well, avoid foods that will make you sick (as much as this may sound like advice that doesn't require retelling, many people routinely eat foods they know will make them sick). Don't give in to food manufacturers' ideas of what you should eat: what's cool, what's in, what will make you richer, have more fun, better looking, or more popular. Stick to foods that support your optimum health. Before you know it, you will have more fun—because you are healthy, energetic, and full of enthusiasm for life.

CHAPTER 3

The Disease Process: How & Why Your Body Breaks Down

What happens when our bodies break down? What happens when we get a cold, when we get cancer, when we get diabetes? How much control do we have over the process of disease? To a great extent, what we put into our bodies, and what we fail to put into our bodies, is responsible for disease. Chronic disease is now felt to be 70% a result of poor nutrition.

Have you ever *known* you were going to come down with a cold, long before you even felt a sniffle or a sore throat? How did you know? Was it because you felt cold for a period of time, or because you had to sit in a damp, cold environment? Did you know that you weren't eating right, that you were missing important nutrients from your diet? Were you aware of stress; did you recognize that you weren't getting enough sleep? Was all of this summed up by you as "feeling a bit run down"? And when this happened, did you try to correct the causes? Did you take a bit of downtime to help your body repair itself? You knew intuitively you were going to "come down with something". Like the busy, stress-filled life that led you to this point, did you write this off as an inevitable result of modern life?

Many of the causes of today's diseases are still not fully understood. Still more are understood (how and why they occur), but we have not yet found a way to correct (cure) the body when it does go wrong. AIDS, many forms of cancer, and multiple sclerosis are all examples. Many of the driving forces behind the disease process are not within our control. It would be nice if we could all live in a clean environment without air, water, or soil pollution. It would be nice if we could find a way to easily control stress in our lives. The reality, however, is far removed from this idyllic picture. The best most of us can do is minimize the toxic effects on our bodies—the ones within our control—and maximize the benefits.

What does all this mean? Well, in a nutshell (you've heard it all before), it means you should eat lots of fresh fruits and vegetables, whole grains, nuts, and seeds. It means you should limit your intake of saturated fats and do your best to eliminate your intake of trans fats. It means "new foods" may have to be eliminated (see more on allergies later in this chapter). New foods include dairy, wheat, soy, and possibly legumes (beans and peas).[1] It means you should limit your intake of sugar. It means you should avoid alcohol, tobacco, and all drugs if at all possible. It means you should exercise moderately, including a program that builds muscle and contains weight-bearing exercise (this last especially important for women to lower the chance of developing osteoporosis). It means you should have *balance* in your life. Balance between work, play, and rest. It means you shouldn't ignore your spiritual side. It means you should laugh a bit, learn to give. It means you should minimize stress *at all costs*.

These are the things within your immediate control. There are other lesser known things you can do to help avoid disease. We'll look at a few in detail to give you a better understanding of what we know and don't know about each of the more prevalent diseases in today's society. Many of our conditions and diseases stem from *affluence*. In the movie "Four Weddings and a Funeral", a 12-year old amateur filmmaker displays a movie he has made of a wedding. He shows happy, elated people dancing, eating, talking. Many of them are very overweight. After these images are ingrained in our minds and we are relaxed, he intersperses images of third world children with their distended bellies and flies crawling in their eyes. It is a stark contrast and certainly an unpleasant comparison, but one that bears thinking about when one considers disease.

Most of us could certainly do well on fewer calories, or at the very least lower caloric concentrations (a slice of cheesecake would be high in caloric concentration—each bite contains far more calories than, say, a slice of whole grain bread). In the introduction, we talked about how in our quest to be thin and "healthy", we have tried to cut all fat out of our diets, but in the process have added more and more sugar and other simple, overprocessed carbohydrates. Confucius claimed that a bowl of rice daily was enough for life[2]. That, and his bended arm for a pillow. It is excess that has driven us to so much disease. And excess continues to drive much of society today, though most of us know better. We have gadgets that cut and chop vegetables, machines that rise bread (no kneading required), garages attached to our houses so that we need never feel real air on our way to work in the morning. When we get to work we park underground and then we take the elevator up to our offices. We have computers, fax machines, modems, cell phones, intercoms, an international postal system, and couriers (for when we're *really* in a hurry). Our bodies have fallen into disuse because of all the "modern conveniences" we have that supposedly make life easier. To compensate, we may get on an electronic treadmill for a half hour while catching up on business news after dinner, but we will probably sit up late working or watching TV, depriving our bodies of yet another essential ingredient to good health—*sleep*. Aside from serious athletes, the people who get the most movement in their lives may be mothers who ferry children around to soccer, baseball, ballet, piano, swimming lessons, and choir. With never a moment to rest, however, what these mothers lack, once again, is *balance*.

What's the answer? There are no easy answers. We can only stress how important it is to find this balance in our lives. Failure to do so can result in serious injury to health. You may not feel the effects of overwork or overweight for many years, perhaps never. However, in all likelihood it will affect the quality of your life and will probably also shorten your life. Do whatever it takes to increase the good in your life and to eliminate the bad.

We need to clarify the word *disease* before we proceed. Many alternative and naturopathic practitioners use the term *dis-ease*, meaning a body that is not at ease with itself or its surroundings. It means something's not right. You could easily argue over the semantics of the word—what is merely a *condition*? What can be considered a *disease*? What is a *health complaint*? The problem with definition is well illustrated by one author who called menopause a disease. Of course it isn't. Menopause is … well, it isn't even a condition. Menopause is a *life process*, like growth or puberty. We wouldn't normally call a life process a disease, or even a condition, would we? For the sake of clarity, we lump all health complaints under the heading "disease" in this book, and only those where the term really doesn't apply, like with menopause, will we make the distinction. Fair enough?

The Disease Process Explained

Allergies

Allergy response is a normal protective device of our own immune system. It can be a friendly reminder or sometimes life-threatening. Most allergies are based on protein in a "lock and key" fit. Common ones we are aware of:

(1) outdoors: bee stings, pollen, moulds, and grasses (hay fever);

(2) indoors: dust mites, moulds;

(3) foods: peanuts, cow's milk, and wheat.

The friendly reminder goes awry with repeated exposure, very large exposure, or if the body's memory is over-acute. An example of this severity is when smell alone triggers a very bad reaction—like the smell of peanuts or fish.

Several choices are available to fine-tune or control the body's immune response. Firstly, avoid the item. Secondly, desensitize the person (not always possible or successful). Thirdly, blunt the body's response with antihistamine or cortisone-like drugs.

You can address allergens a number of ways, but first you have to find the source of the allergens. If the allergens are in the environment or your home, you might consider relocating to a different city/georgraphic area or moving to a different house. If allergens are occupational, changes you could make include performing some other kind of work or avoiding workplace allergens (for instance, a surgical nurse sensitive to latex can use non-latex gloves). Reducing the level and number of allergens is often a great help if big changes are not possible.

A careful history is still the mainstay of health practitioners. Food allergies are evaluated by elimination diets as the gold standard. Skin injections of food allergens are fraught with problems and are quite unreliable. Today we can choose ELISA as a blood test to indicate our sensitivities ($300-400), or electrodermal testing.

Dr. Bill Code:

> I suggest electrodermal testing by an experienced health practitioner. I found several food and chemical sensitivities I was unaware of and believe this to be another step taken toward wellness.

Body responses to allergens are varied, and include skin rashes and eczema (*dermatitis*). Emu oil is both immediately soothing to these and often therapeutic. Acute asthma or breathing difficulty is a life-threatening emergency and needs to be handled in an emergency room. Education, including comprehensive sensitivity testing and evaluation by your health care professional, is key in follow-up. If foods are a significant component—and they often are—then education and diet changes by a skilled dietician are very useful.

Asthma and the spasms of the lung muscles that cause the "starving for air" that sufferers describe, is a result of chronic inflammation and hypersensitivity of the lungs and airway passages to certain stimuli. Asthma specialists tell us that rising levels of environmental pollutants are the reason for the rise in asthma cases and the severity of them. A host of attack-provoking allergens have been identified.

Common allergens include hairspray, perfumes, dust, animal dander, pollen, mould spores, chemicals, dust mites, drugs, food additives such as sulfites, and food allergies such as milk or wheat. Occupational allergens include chemicals such as urethane and polyurethane (used in the manufacture of plastics and glues) and dry cleaning chemicals. Common irritants to our airways (breathing tubes) are tobacco smoke and fumes such as paints or smog (a word made from "smoke" and "fog"). Note— this list is incomplete and only certain allergens affect certain people (for example, while you may be allergic to the particles in hairspray, you may tolerate milk perfectly well).

Eczema is a condition characterized by an inflammatory response of the skin causing redness, itching, minute blisters, weeping, oozing, and crusting. It is a common allergic reaction in children, but also affects adults. It is thought that food sensitivities and a lack of essential fatty acids (including polyunsaturated fatty acids) contributes to the development of this condition. You will read more about eczema in Chapter 9.

Autoimmune Diseases

"Auto" means "self" (think *autonomy)*. Paired with "immune" it literally means immune to one's self. All the conditions and diseases under this heading have one thing in common—they are all the result of an overzealous immune system. Somewhere, as a trigger, a partially digested protein snuck past the gut's entry (i.e., *leaky gut)* and the liver's neutralizing enzymes and has made its way into our immune system. It has been suggested, for instance, that juvenile onset diabetes (insulin-dependent diabetes) begins with an allergy to cow's milk. Undigested whey protein gets into a child's body and the immune system responds by attacking it. The "immune soldiers" are now trained to recognize this foreign invader, and to be "on alert." They will attack each time this "foreign" protein enters the body. However, the antibodies against the milk protein may be only slightly altered and now attack the body's own proteins in the pancreatic cells that produce insulin.

This is how autoimmune diseases start. Which cells in the body the antibodies attack is dependent on which cells they tend to mimic. If whey proteins tend to mimic pancreatic protein cells, then diabetes may result. Other self-mimicking proteins are soy, wheat, and corn. These proteins are often ones changed in the last fifty years in search of an "ideal" product to sell.

It is advisable, of course, if such a reaction to a type or class of food is noted, to avoid the food completely. When the food is first consumed, "allergic reactions" may be the visible result. However, repeated assaults to the immune system with the allergen may result in the protein mimicking proteins in the body, in which case the body eventually turns on itself, as explained in the example of diabetes. In the case of multiple sclerosis, the body attacks the myelin sheath (in the brain and spinal cord), the protective and insulating coating around nerve cells.

Autoimmune diseases are considered to be "society's" diseases. The food we eat, the schedules we keep, the sleep we lack, and the environments in which we live, all contribute to the body's immune system sometimes going into overdrive and eventually turning on itself. Society's diseases used to mean sexually transmitted ones like syphilis, gonorrhea and herpes!

Chronic Fatigue Syndrome is also called an *energy* disease because it seems to affect the mitochondria of cells, where *metabolism* of cell matter (making energy from carbon fuels) takes place.

Fibromyalgia is another condition sometimes known as an energy disease. Neither chronic fatigue syndrome nor fibromyalgia are well understood and most so-called "yuppie" flu conditions—that is, general malaise, low energy, chronic achiness, and fatigue symptoms—are lumped into one of these two categories. Fibromyalgia is implicated in cases where there appears to be soft tissue pain that can be identified as being attributed to several specific areas of the body.

Inflammatory Bowel Diseases - Please see under "Gastrointestinal Diseases".

Multiple Sclerosis is a disease in which the body's immune system attacks the myelin—the fatty protective coating around nerves in the brain and spinal cord. This attacking of the cells creates a secondary response which causes inflammation, swelling, pain, and loss of use of the affected areas. MS is characterized by a wide range of symptoms, and the difficulty with it is that no two cases are alike, nor can the progression of the disease be predicted. Many common symptoms include abnormal sensations such as burning, tingling, or prickling in the face, head, arms, hands, legs, or feet. Muscle weakness or unusual tiring of an arm or leg, stiffness, gait disturbances like foot drop, loss of bladder control, vertigo (dizziness), and emotional disturbances can also occur. Nausea and vomiting, slurred speech, tremors, difficulty breathing and, for men, impotence, are other common symptoms. As the disease progresses, a person with MS may have a staggering gait. In advanced stages of the disease, movement may become erratic and chronic urinary incontinence or urgency may occur. Extreme or a vague, all-over fatigue is present in most cases of MS and present through almost all flare-ups. Stress, certain foods, and excessive environmental heat can make MS symptoms worse.

Dr. Bill Code:

> As you may remember from the prologue, I was diagnosed with multiple sclerosis at age 42. Today, there are more diet-based changes that can help control MS for many people. Dr. Swank's low fat diet is a consideration. I believe all fats that aren't essential fatty acids should be minimized. I no longer eat deep-fried foods or hydrogenated vegetable oils. Food allergies (e.g., wheat and dairy products) are likely involved. Finally, increased vitamin D, a recognized body hormone which modulates the immune system, may prevent progression. Why are multiple sclerosis and inflammatory bowel diseases so common in Canada? A deficiency in vitamin D may be one of the reasons.

Osteoarthritis is a form of arthritis with major incapacity, loss of work, and disability. It involves deterioration of the cartilage that covers the ends of the bones—typically the knees, tips of fingers, joints of the spine, and hips (especially in men). Joints develop knobbiness. Once thought to be a "wear and tear" disease associated with aging, it is now thought that autoimmunity plays a role. There is a breakdown of cartilage and lack of collagen and synovial fluid—the substances within joints that attract and hold water and work to cushion the bones from one another as a person moves. *Gouty arthritis*, affecting mostly males over the age of 40, usually affects the big toe, but occasionally other joints as well. Onset of gout is sudden and causes extreme pain.

Another serious condition known as *Raynaud's phenomenon* involves constriction and spasm of the blood vessels in extremities: fingers, toes, and the tip of the nose. The disease affects mostly women and can lead to gangrene in extreme cases. It is usually an autoimmune disease, so diet, nutritional needs, and food allergies can all be involved.

Psoriasis is a condition characterized by patches of silvery scales or red areas on the skin. It is often hereditary and is linked to rapid growth of cells in the skin's outer layer. Psoriasis is hardly known in countries where diets are low in fat, and in fact may be the result of the body's incorrectly metabolizing, or faulty utilization, of fat. Lowering trans and saturated fats in the diet is indicated, as well as making sure enough essential fatty acids are included in the diet, with supplementation called for in most cases. Recent research points to evidence that psoriasis is an autoimmune condition. Emu oil always helps the itch and burn of psoriasis. In addition, it will resolve some cases, and in others enhance other medications as a carrier and/or as a synergistic agent.

Rheumatoid Arthritis and **Juvenile Rheumatoid Arthritis** are other types of inflammatory arthritis. It is an autoimmune disorder (a self attacking self) disease, in which the body's immune system improperly identifies the synovial membranes that secrete the lubricating fluid in the joints as foreign. The result is inflammation and the cartilage and tissues in bone surfaces are destroyed as well. It can occur at any age, but the peak incidence of disease onset is between the ages of 25 and 55. Women are affected three times more often than men. The incidence increases with age, and approximately 3% of the population is affected. The course and the severity of the illness can vary considerably.

The onset of the disease is usually slow, with fatigue, loss of appetite, weakness, and vague muscular symptoms. Eventually, joint pain appears, with warmth, swelling, tenderness, and stiffness after inactivity of the joint. Suggestions of topical comfort and slowing progression can be found in Chapters 6, 9, and 11.

Systemic Lupus Erythematosus (SLE) occurs primarily in women (9:1 ratio). SLE is felt to be an autoimmune disease. Our immune system is attacking our blood vessels (vasculitis) in potentially many different body regions. This includes skin, heart, lungs, the gastrointestinal tract, kidneys, joints, and the brain. SLE has a genetic risk of about 10%. Once again, the best treatment is prevention. Vitamin D at 1,000 IU daily to prevent, and up to 4,000 IU per day to enhance immune system modulation if SLE is already present. If *prednisone* and other steroids are in use, vitamin D, calcium, and magnesium will slow the upcoming osteoporosis.

Recurrent or Chronic
Infectious and Viral Diseases

Acne - The skin contains oil-producing structures called pilosebaceous follicles, which are present in large quantities on the face, chest, shoulders, and upper back. Each of these follicles consists of a hair follicle and a sebaceous gland. The glands secrete an oily mixture called sebum which normally passes through the hair follicle to the skin surface. Acne occurs when the normal route of sebum to the skin surface is blocked by dead skin cells, bacteria, hormones, and extra oil. The obstruction leads to swelling and the development of blackheads, whiteheads, or tender red lumps (pimples). It was once thought that poor hygiene or over-consumption of certain foods—particularly chocolate—were to blame for acne. We now know these are not causes. Emotional stress, fatigue, humidity, and certain cosmetics may aggravate acne. You will hear more about acne control in the chapter on skin care.

AIDS – Though we don't think of AIDS as an infectious disease, that's how it's contracted—from one infected person to another. Body fluids like blood or semen must be exchanged in order for the disease to pass from one person to another. Sharing of plates, cutlery, and glasses will not spread AIDS. HIV must be present in a person before AIDS can set in, though not all people who are HIV-positive will develop the disease; some (though a small percentage) never do. Once AIDS does become active, the body loses its ability to fight off common diseases or their effects. Examples would be flus, pneumonia, herpes, *Epstein-Barr* virus (the virus that causes infectious mononucleosis and may contribute to chronic fatigue syndrome), and tuberculosis.

Cold Sores start as small ulcerations in the mouth and on the lips. They look like little pimples—they have white centres and red, inflamed borders and are very painful. Women tend to get these more than men. They'll heal on their own within 10-14 days, but in the meantime can cause a lot of aggravation and have a tendency to flare up in multiples and also to recur.

Colds – Ah, yes, the common cold. We still haven't found a cure, of course. You can do *so much* to help prevent the onset of a cold, or to speed recovery and lessen the severity of symptoms when you do get one. No need to describe the symptoms—you all know what they are.

How to avoid getting a cold:
• Eat right: lots of fresh fruits and vegetables;

- Exercise moderately;
- Avoid nasty things like cigarette smoke, coffee, alcohol, drugs;
- Limit the amount of simple starches, bad fats, and sugar— empty calories—you consume;
- Drink lots of fluids, especially water. You should drink 8-10 glasses of pure (distilled or reverse osmosis) water every day;
- Take vitamins and minerals according to our supplementation recommendations in Chapter 6, especially Vitamins C, D, E, beta carotene, potassium (though you'll get lots of this if you follow the next step religiously), and zinc;
- Take two tablespoons of apple cider vinegar (the raw kind you buy in opaque bottles at your health food store) in half a glass of tepid water every morning on an empty stomach;[3]
- Get plenty of fresh air every day. If it's cold or rainy out, then dress accordingly;
- Increase consumption of garlic and onions. Garlic is one of the most potent *natural* antibiotic and antioxidant substances available;
- Avoid stress at all costs. Stress eventually compromises the immune system's ability to fight off infection;
- Get lots of rest and plenty of sleep. The average person needs at least nine hours sleep per night (don't laugh, thinking you could never get this much—*find a way*... it is vital to your health);
- Humidifiers in your living room, bedroom, and office can help keep the membranes of the upper respiratory tract moist; and
- Keep your hands clean. Wash them often, especially when you have been in public places like stores, restaurants, and public transit.

When you do get a cold, here's what you can do to speed up recovery:

- Eat lots of fruit and drink lots of fruit juice;
- Take three to four times the vitamin C recommended in Chapter 6 (should be in the range of 3-4 grams). Also make sure you are getting plenty of zinc, vitamin E, and beta carotene (beta carotene is safe to take in larger doses for short periods of time, whereas vitamin A can be toxic, particularly if you are pregnant. Again, check our chart for daily allowances and toxicity ranges);
- Drink lots of water and plain, *unsweetened* herbal teas. There are good mixtures available at your health food store designed specifically to help you if you have a cold;
- Rest. Rest. Rest;
- Certain herbs and natural supplements work wonders to speed recovery. Echinacea has become very popular. Use as soon as you feel run down. Look for combination formulas that contain both *echinacea angustifolia* and *echinacea purpurea.* Do not use any herbs continuously—therapeutic use should be limited to a few weeks at a time. Other useful herbs are golden seal, cayenne (*capsaicin*), garlic, wild cherry bark, and ginger;
- Avoid over-the-counter medications like antihistamines and nasal sprays. While these may help symptoms in the short-term, they may actually lengthen the duration of your cold. Any drugs that work by drying out your membranes usually dry them out too much and have the reverse effect—this makes it *harder* for your body to fight the infection it has. Overuse or misuse of nasal sprays will also backfire on you. You will end up with *increasing* nasal congestion and possibly a chronic problem; and
- Even if you have a *flu* (fever, vomiting, diarrhea), you should stay away from antibiotics. Both colds and flus are viral infections and will not be helped by antibiotics, which are designed to kill *bacteria*, not *viruses*. Sometimes, a secondary *bacterial infection* develops and then antibiotics are indicated.

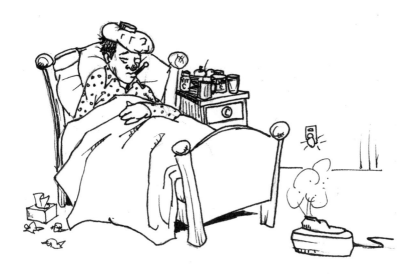

These infections are of the respiratory tract, the stomach and intestines or, in the case of pneumonia, the lungs. However, in most circumstances, a flu need only be investigated if it has held on for more than two weeks. At this time, the doctor will look for a bacterial infection. Antibiotics will do more harm than good when taken for the common flu and cold.

If you take antibiotics for a cold, two things happen that you don't want. First of all, broad spectrum antibiotics do not just kill the offending bacteria in your system, they kill *all* the bacteria in your system, including the friendly bacteria we told you about in the discussion about your digestion. When you mis- or overuse broad spectrum antibiotics, your body loses its ability to fight off other infections, because it is partly the good bacteria in your system that does this. The result is increased risk of many types of infections, including *fungal* or *viral* infections that will lead to flu or other conditions with flu-like symptoms.

With antibiotic use, the second thing that happens is that your body may be finding a way to fight—or resist—that particular antibiotic. Especially with the overuse of antibiotics, bacteria can find a way to "outsmart" the antibiotic. When this happens, you end up with *stronger* and more *potent* bad bacteria in your body, better able to withstand antibiotic treatment. You don't want this when you really *do* have a bad bacterial infection like meningitis. We already have increasing antibiotic resistance due to the presence of antibiotics in animal feeds, and by extension in the animal foods we consume.

Herpes is a common viral infection that causes cold sores and genital sores. You will read much more about herpes in our chapter on skin care. Avoid foods such as chocolate, bad fats, sugars, refined carbohydrates, coffee, and tea. Remember that stress can precipitate outbreaks and make them more severe.

Urinary Tract Infections, which include bladder infections and in extreme cases kidney disease, are infectious diseases caused by different bacterias, the most common of which is E. coli. As with any infectious disease, it is wise to supplement with *good bacteria*, such as *lactobacillus acidophilus, B. bifidus,* and others, found in blended capsules in the refrigerated section of your health food store.

You can also get these beneficial bacteria by eating yogurt, but many commercially prepared yogurts do not have anywhere near the active bacterial content you want. What you are looking for is bacteria that is still alive, not sterile as it likely is with many supermarket-type brands. Buy your yogurt at the health food store. You'll pay a little more, but the benefits are really worth the price difference.

Yogurt is also an excellent way to get calcium, especially if you have problems with lactose-containing foods. In yogurt, the lactose has been mostly pre-digested and so does not cause the same symptoms as milk might. And there's more good news with yogurt: low fat yogurt has more calcium than milk (452 mg calcium per cup vs. 275 mg calcium per cup) and also more calcium than whole milk yogurt, because they add more milk solids to achieve that rich creaminess that makes it taste more like whole milk yogurt. This makes yogurt an excellent choice when viewed from all health angles, and particularly if you are trying to limit dietary fat (especially from animal products).

Your doctor may decide the best course of action for your urinary tract infection (UTI) is antibiotics. This would certainly be called for if the infection travels up the urinary tract and reaches your kidneys. If this happens you could develop kidney disease, which of course is to be avoided at all costs. Again, an ounce of prevention is worth a pound of cure. Good hygiene (remember, wipe from front to back!), proper bacteria balance in the body (which you can help achieve and maintain with a proper diet and, at times, supplements), natural clothing that does not fit too tightly, are all excellent ways to help combat this condition. One of the most beneficial dietary items you can consume if you have a chronic problem with UTIs is cranberry juice. Cranberry juice tablets are available at health food stores, but like so many foods-versus-supplements arguments, researchers have found that consuming just a small quantity of the *pure* juice every day (not the *cocktail* which contains little cranberry juice and lots of sugar) is much more beneficial than taking the capsules. Again, it is the synergy of the active ingredients in cranberry juice together with the other components in the juice that likely make it so effective.

Yeast Infections – Much was said about yeast infections or *Candida albicans* several years ago. Everything was said to cause it—too much starch, too much sugar, too much fruit—you name it. Oral contraceptives can lead to a higher incidence of yeast infections, as can pregnancy—when the balance of sugars and hormones in a woman's body alters. Again, an acidophilus product or yogurt containing live bacterial culture is the best defense and the best treatment. Yeast infections are often a problem when a woman overuses or misuses antibiotics, as you'll remember from *colds and flus*. If you cannot avoid taking a course of broad spectrum antibiotics, start immediately on a course of acidophilus, staying on it at least two weeks to one month after you have finished the antibiotic treatment.

Endocrine Diseases

Your endocrine system is the system of glands in the body, including the thyroid, adrenals, parathyroid, endocrine glands of the pancreas, and pituitary. These glands secrete hormones whose purpose is to evoke a specific response to cells of the body, cells which are often far away from the gland itself. The hormones are released into the bloodstream, and the blood then carries them to the site at which they are needed.

The most commonly known endocrine disorder is diabetes mellitus, in which the glands of the pancreas cease to secrete certain hormones. Two of these are insulin and glucagon, which are vital in controlling the body's blood sugar.

Common Disorders of the Thyroid

The *thyroid gland* is the largest gland in the neck, shaped somewhat like a bow tie. It is at the front of your neck, protected by layers of muscle and skin. The thyroid's primary function is to make the thyroid hormone, which has an effect on nearly all tissues of the body, where it increases cellular activity. Therefore, the thyroid can be seen to control and regulate the body's metabolism. The two most common disorders of the thyroid are *hyper*thyroidism and *hypo*thyroidism. *Hyper* is defined as *too much*, which means that the thyroid is creating too much of the thyroid hormone. *Hypo* is defined as *too little:* the thyroid creates too little of the thyroid hormone.

Other thyroid problems include goiter, cancer (though growths or tumours on the thyroid can also be benign), and thyroiditis, which is an autoimmune inflammatory process and usually leads to hypothyroidism.

The *parathyroid glands* are small glands located behind the thyroid. There are four of them, each about the size of a pea; their normal color is that of mustard. The primary purpose of the parathyroid glands is to regulate the calcium levels in our bodies within a very narrow range so that the nervous and muscular systems can function properly. Although they are neighbours (geographically speaking) and are both part of the endocrine system, the parathyroid glands and thyroid gland are otherwise unrelated. The most common diseases of the parathyroid glands are over- or under-production of the parathyroid hormones, causing a potentially serious calcium imbalance.

The *pancreas* is basically a digestive organ but it also has two very important hormonal functions. It produces the pancreatic endocrine hormones *insulin* and *glucagon*. These hormones help regulate many aspects of our metabolism, the most well-known being that of blood sugar. The pancreas' other function is to produce pancreatic digestive enzymes.

The digestive, or enzyme secretion portion of the pancreas makes up more than 90 per cent of its total cell mass. The digestive (or exocrine) pancreas is responsible for making digestive enzymes which are secreted into the intestines to help digest the food we eat. These enzymes digest proteins, fats, and carbohydrates into much smaller molecules (see the chapter on digestion), so that our intestines can absorb them.

The endocrine portion of the pancreas is the one that makes the hormones that regulate sugar levels in the blood. These endocrine cells are clustered in groups within the pancreas which look like little islands of cells when examined under a microscope. This led to these groups of cells being named "Pancreatic Islets." Within the islets are cells which make the hormones we've been talking about, the most famous of which, of course, is insulin. These cells are called "Pancreatic Islet Cells" or *Islets of Langerhans.*

The two main glucose controlling hormones are: *insulin* and *glucagon.* Insulin lowers blood sugar and is secreted in response to high blood glucose. Glucagon has the opposite action and is secreted in response to low blood glucose.

Diabetes is a serious and potentially life-threatening degenerative disease characterized by the body no longer producing insulin, or producing too little. Though we can certainly term it as an endocrine disorder (because there is a malfunctioning organ), it can also be classified as an autoimmune disease as the body's immune system, for some reason, attacks the Islet of Langerhans cells that produce insulin in the pancreas.

Type I Diabetes is usually juvenile onset (onset in young people). Very little or no insulin is produced by the pancreas. These people need to inject insulin under the skin several times a day. The amount of insulin and frequency of injections is determined by finger pokes for blood and a glucometer (a small machine with digital readout). A diabetic's education on how best to control his or her condition is important and is best undertaken by a team of dietician, nurse, and physician.

Type II Diabetes is "maturity onset" and is increasingly common (up to 7% of Canadians). It is primarily insulin resistance by our bodies. Increased body fat increases our insulin resistance. This insulin resistance of cells causes more insulin to be secreted, which usually increases our body fat. This is a vicious cycle. The only way off the merry-go-round is whole foods, increased fiber, reduced caloric intake, and gradual weight loss.

Certainly, simple sugars, simple carbohydrates, and refined foods head us toward disaster. Principles in the weight loss chapter should be reviewed. Some people have found improved blood sugar control by taking 3-5 emu oil capsules per day.

Gallbladder Disease - The gallbladder is a small organ located directly under the liver. It acts as a reservoir for bile and concentrates bile. Bile, a combination of cholesterol, bile salts, lecithin, and other substances, is secreted by the liver and is used by the body to digest fats. Gallbladder difficulties are very common in North America. The first sign of a problem is often colicky pain after a meal high in fat or one consumed when under emotional stress. The pain is in the right side of the ribcage (above the abdomen) and often radiates around the side and to the upper back between the shoulder blades. Attacks range from mild to excruciating and can last from 20 minutes to several hours. A severe attack is characterized by nausea, vomiting, and fever. Acute, severe gallbladder attacks must be addressed immediately. If they are not, inflammation and infection of the gallbladder can result, and this can be life threatening.

Gallstone formation is the result of many years of a high fat diet and also of lifestyle, and are common in people who lose weight quickly. Gallstones which are small or that resemble gravel-like sludge are reversible; stones of 0.5 cm (1/3 inch) in diameter or more are not. Many people simply opt to have the gallbladder removed. While many will tell you that the gallbladder is an unnecessary organ, it does have a function. It releases bile to help digest fats, and after an especially fatty meal, this is very important. It also stores bile, and therefore there is more of it for the body to use in the digestive process, as compared to the body relying solely on the bile present in the liver. However, it is also important to address the presence of gallstones.

Hypoglycemia is the opposite to hyperglycemia. This is a fairly common condition. It happens when there is an over-production of insulin, which results in not enough glucose in the bloodstream. Another cause of hypoglycemia is when there is an under-production of the hormone glucagon, which is the hormone that signals the liver to release glucose into the bloodstream. Hypoglycemia is not difficult to control. Vigilant attention to regular meals (sometimes smaller, more frequent meals are called for), and attention to the right types of foods will often be enough to control this condition.

The most important aspect of a good diet for the person prone to hypoglycemia is to limit or eliminate simple sugars like candy, cake, and pop, and to be cautious with foods like mashed potatoes, bagels, pancakes, and other innocuous seeming foods. Some of these foods are absorbed into the bloodstream incredibly quickly, leaving room for the inevitable sugar crash that follows about an hour later. If you are prone to hypoglycemia, consume whole grain products, always include protein (and *good* fats) with your meals and snacks, and ensure that your carbohydrates contain plenty of fiber. The fiber is more extensive in whole foods, and it helps moderate the glucose rise in the bloodstream. This rapid glucose rise or spike results in increased insulin, which drives down blood sugar.

Kidney Stones are believed to develop when substances in the urine form crystals that cling together. Stones are usually only a fraction of an inch in diameter and surfaces may be smooth or jagged. There are numerous reasons why stones may develop. If a person is chronically dehydrated, the amount of fluid in the urine can drop, so that stone-forming substances in it become unusually concentrated. Excessive calcium in the blood can result from bone degeneration that releases calcium into the bloodstream, from excessive absorption of calcium from the gastrointestinal tract (which can result from overactive parathyroid glands), or from increased reabsorption from the kidneys.[4]

Best decisions for prevention of kidney stones are based on having your own stone analyzed for content. About 75% are of calcium salts. Some 10% of stones occur as the result of bladder infection. Another 10% are from uric acid (of gouty arthritis fame), and about 2% are of cysteine (an amino acid). The final 2-3% are of many and assorted types, often secondary to drug therapy. The only universal concept is drink more water (8-10 glasses per day—see our discussion about water in Chapter 2). Current concept for calcium stones is increasing your calcium intake, especially at bedtime. Most of these people are removing calcium from their bones! Calcium loss from "bones into stones" is worsened by carbonated beverages, due to their high phosphorus content. Vitamin D supplementation is best avoided in this case. Follow-up by a urologist or endocrinologist is best considered. Bladder infection merits careful treatment and follow-up. If simple measures are ineffective, see an expert.

Osteoporosis is a progressive, degenerative disease in which the bones become weak and brittle (*osteo* means bone and *porosis* refers to porousness or "airiness"), and prone to breakage. The disease affects more women than men and is more prevalent than heart disease, stroke, diabetes, breast cancer, or arthritis. You will often see an elderly person with a very humped back—this is a result of bones in the spinal cord which have literally crumbled away. This leaves the spine with less to hold it upright, thus forming the familiar "curvature." Best efforts on osteoporosis are on prevention. Vitamin D_3: 1,000 units per day (see chapter on dietary supplements) with 1,200 mgs of calcium. If osteoporosis has been diagnosed, take 4,000 IU daily of Vitamin D_3 and 1,500 mg of calcium. Make sure your formula also contains magnesium. The magnesium in the product should be half that of the calcium. These measures will slow the progression of osteoporosis dramatically and may even partly reverse the condition. Reduced hip fractures is an important goal. Why? Because 50% of the time, people with broken hips end up losing their life independence.

Women's Health Issues

Menopause is not a disease. Instead, it is a life process marked by decreases in the production of certain hormones. It is, of course, the time of life when a woman's monthly periods cease and her child-bearing years come to an end. At this time, the hormone estrogen is produced in much lower amounts than before and this causes changes in all kinds of areas: metabolism, maintenance of stable body temperature, and calcium balance in the body. It can affect sleep patterns and mood, and there may be changes in sexual function—vaginal dryness and decreased libido.

There are wonderful books available to help women cope with the "change of life." Diet, exercise, and frame of mind play a big role in severity of symptoms. Women are encouraged to see menopause as a time of celebration—entering the "wise woman" years. This can be done with regret, or it can be done with grace.

Essential fatty acids and soy products (which have estrogen-like effects) are two of the most effective additions to the diet a woman can make to help minimize the undesirable effects of menopause. Issues of skin or vaginal dryness can be eased with emu oil. Plant based estrogens and progesterones, applied topically with emu oil or *liposomes*, are often better tolerated than *Premarin* (the pharmaceutical product made from pregnant horse urine) or similar synthetics.

Premenstrual Syndrome is a hormonal condition which can be helped with essential fatty acids, particularly omega-3 fatty acids. Diet and exercise also play a big role in helping to minimize the symptoms of PMS. Vitamin B6 and magnesium deficiencies have been linked to severe symptoms, so supplementation of these may be beneficial. Caffeine, sugar, a diet high in simple carbohydrates, and stress may make symptoms worse. Many women have found comfort in an emu oil-based warm rub massaged on the lower abdomen.

Neurological Disorders

Many neurological disorders may have their roots in poor energy transfer between cells, or impaired or compromised nerve activity. In the brain, the millions of cells (composed 50% of fatty acids) depend on impulses (like electrical charges) which send messages back and forth. When those nerve pathways are damaged, or there are insufficient nutrients like essential fatty acids to repair and rebuild cells, impaired function results. The combination of a lack of essential fatty acids and the need to control inflammation in so many neurological and autoimmune conditions makes emu oil a fine addition to any health regimen. There will be more about this in the chapters on emu oil.

Alzheimer's Disease (AD) is a condition characterized by impaired mental function. At first, symptoms begin slowly, and the only symptom may be mild forgetfulness. It has been said, however, that if you are aware of your forgetfulness, it is simply normal forgetfulness; if you are unaware of it, it could be the early stages of AD. People with AD may have trouble remembering recent events, activities, or the names of familiar people or things. Simple math problems may become difficult to solve.

As the disease progresses, symptoms are more easily noticed and become serious enough to cause people to seek medical help. For example, AD sufferers may forget how to do simple tasks, like brushing their teeth or combing their hair. They can no longer think clearly, and they begin to have problems speaking, understanding, reading, or writing. Later on, people with

AD may become anxious or aggressive, or wander away from home. Eventually, patients may need total care.

Studies show that supplementation with vitamin E (d-alpha-tocopherol acetate) is now considered a vital and common part of treatment in the early stages of AD. While cognition (brain function) may not improve, supplementation at this level has been proven to slow degeneration and decline.[5] Even patients with mild AD are now urged to take 2,000 IU of vitamin E daily. This report adds that patients with vitamin K and clotting abnormalities should not take vitamin E at this dose, and instead should stick to the recommended level of 800-1,000 IU.

Other supplementation recommended is ginkgo biloba, which has been prescribed for sufferers of AD for many years now, particularly in Europe. It has the effect of dilating blood vessels and increasing circulation, particularly to the brain.

A 1997 study reported in the *Journal of the American Medical Association* showed symptomatic and cognitive improvement with the use of ginkgo biloba. Of 309 patients, 27% showed improvement, compared with 14% taking a placebo. On another measurable scale, 37% were considered improved, compared with 23% taking a placebo. The treatment was considered safe and no adverse side effects were reported.[6]

The Neurobiology of Aging February 16, 2000 issue reports that anti-inflammatory agents may be of some use in patients with AD. This report covered non-steroidal anti-inflammatory drugs (NSAIDs) like Ibuprofen. Remember, however, that NSAIDs worsen leaky gut syndrome. A safer anti-inflammatory could be emu oil gel capsules.

Carpal Tunnel Syndrome affects a large proportion of the population (about 3% of adults). There is pain, numbness, and/or tingling in the hand from the thumb to the ring finger. Risk factors include being female, obesity, employment in blue-collar occupations, and using excessive force with the hand or working with excessive wrist flexion or extension while on the job. The inflammation that results can be addressed with emu oil being rubbed on the arm several times a day. Supplementation with vitamin B6 should be considered, but under a health practitioner's care, as toxicity can occur. If emu oil by itself is not enough, look for a warm rub of emu oil where other herbs act in synergy.

Depression is not simply a "state of mind". It is not something a person can snap out of any more than a person can snap out of having a flu or pre-menstrual syndrome. Studies have shown a definite link between depression and the brain chemicals serotonin and melatonin. A definite link also exists between depression and nutrition. B-complex vitamins, essential fatty acids, and other vitamins such as vitamin D_3 are essential. When depression strikes, it is important to try to stay involved, get out of doors, and to try to maintain positive, optimistic thoughts. Stress can aggravate depression. Daily exercise such as walking, hiking, or swimming is strongly encouraged. Food sensitivities or allergies may make depression worse. Increase consumption of whole and unprocessed foods, fresh fruits, and vegetables.

Hyperactivity may be seen as being the opposite to depression in some ways. It is characterized by an inability to concentrate or focus on one task at a time. It impairs learning and judgment in both children and adults. While children seem to suffer from hyperactivity more than adults, it is possible that adults are simply more able to put forward a calm outward appearance, making it seem that they are calm, when in fact they are not. *Attention Deficit-Hyperactivity Disorder (ADHD)* in children is being over-medicated with pharmaceutical products such as *Ritalin*. It is advisable, if a child appears to suffer with ADHD, to look very closely at food allergies and nutritional deficiencies. These are often the cause of this disorder. There are supplements available to help calm the ADHD child. One of the more important nutritional supplements to address are essential fatty acids, especially omega-3, i.e., alpha-linolenic acid (ALA).

Migraine Headaches are "vascular" headaches which involve the blood vessels supplying the brain. These blood vessels are excessively dilated or constricted and the resulting spasms cause pain. There are two types of migraine, common and classic. The common migraine occurs slowly, producing a throbbing pain that may last from two to 24 hours. The pain is severe and is often centered at the temple or behind one ear. Alternatively, it can begin at the back of the head and spread to one entire side of the head. It can be accompanied by nausea, vomiting, blurred vision, or tingling and numbness in the limbs.

A classic migraine is similar to a common migraine, but is preceded by a set of symptoms referred to as an *aura*, which can consist of speech disorders, weakness, and disturbances in vision or smell. An aura can also consist of brilliant stars, sparks, flashes, or geometric forms passing across the visual field. The most common symptom is an inability to see clearly. Visual disturbances may last a few seconds or may persist for hours, then disappear.

Doctors and other health professionals offer varying theories on what causes migraine headaches—genetics, low blood sugar (usually the result of a diet rich in sugar and refined starches and low in vitamins and minerals), tension, grief, rage, disappointment, anxiety, liver trouble, constipation (with resulting autointoxication), or possibly allergies to preservatives and to chemical additives in food.

There are some very effective herbs—for example feverfew, white willow bark (equivalent to ASA), valerian, ginkgo biloba, and ginger—that may help the migraine sufferer.

Dr. Bill Code:
> I have found food allergies a major trigger of symptoms of my MS. If I avoid wheat, milk, and orange

juice, I rarely experience headaches. Apparently, 80% of people with MS suffer from migraines—perhaps this is an important clue.

Cardiovascular Diseases

Atherosclerosis and **Arteriosclerosis** involve the buildup of deposits on the insides of the artery walls, which causes thickening and hardening of the arteries. These deposits consist mostly of fatty substances. "Hardening" or thickening of the arteries raises blood pressure—which can also lead to heart attacks or strokes. Most people affected by cardiovascular diseases have at least one risk factor playing a prominent role in their lives—family history of the disease, smoking, high blood pressure, or elevated cholesterol levels. Some have more than one risk factor, and it is important to address this issue. Heart attacks and strokes are still the #1 and #3 causes of death, respectively, in North America.

The most effective way to reduce your risk of developing heart disease is to eliminate or minimize risk factors. If you have high cholesterol, there are natural ways to reduce your cholesterol levels. The best way is to ensure that your diet is not only low in cholesterol and saturated fats, but especially low in trans fats. Avoid everything with "hydrogenated vegetable oil" in it. This includes hard margarines, commercial cookies, breads and baked goods, and definitely deep-fried foods. Your diet should also contain substances known to reduce levels of "bad" cholesterol. Making sure you get plenty of essential fatty acids is one of the most important things you can do. Herbs that improve circulation are listed under *Migraine Headaches*. Another herb excellent for circulation is cayenne pepper, which is available in capsule form.

Additional risk factors should be eliminated—stop smoking, lose weight, and take regular, moderate exercise under the direction of a physician. Within two years of quitting smoking, your heart attack risk is equal to non-smokers. Smokers, on average, die eight years earlier! Controlling levels of stress is also very important in the management of these diseases.

Heart Attack and **Vascular Disease**

Heart attack is the layman's term for *myocardial infarction* (MI). When an MI happens, the heart muscle loses most or all of its blood supply. This blockage is either local plaques (atherosclerosis), embolism (piece of plaque or clot from elsewhere), blood clot at the blockage (thrombosis), or a combination thereof. Treatment includes dissolving the clot very quickly (emergency room TPA or streptokinase), flattening the plaque (angioplasty balloon), or bypass the area (coronary artery bypass surgery). Similar blood vessel problems occur in the abdomen and limbs—all of them are best prevented—as treatment is usually too late for great success.

Nutritional solutions include Dr. Dean Ornishe's challenging approach (less than 10% fats, exercise, and stress reduction) or Dr. Edward N. Siguel's discussion, *Essential Fatty Acids in Health & Disease*. We (the authors) prefer the concepts of the latter. Almost all of us need more omega-3 fatty acids (see ground flax in Chapter 6). We also need to eliminate trans fatty acids (hydrogenated vegetable oils) and reduce our total caloric intake.

Eating primarily whole foods will reduce simple and refined carbohydrates and saturated fats as well. The increased fiber from more fruits, vegetables, legumes, and whole grains will lower cholesterol and low density lipoproteins (both are bad if levels are high).

Elevated *homocysteine levels* are also implicated in heart disease. Read about lowering homocysteine levels under Folic Acid (vitamin B4) in Chapter 6. The issues of stress reduction are addressed in Chapter 5. Chelation therapy is an option for people with no other options available to them.

Dr. Bill Code:

> I had intravenous chelation for heavy metal toxicity (in my case it was lead). Even regular medical textbooks support it for heavy metal poisoning (lead, mercury, cadmium, arsenic, etc.).

Stroke, the number three killer in North America, is quite similar to heart attack. It is a part of the brain losing its blood supply. All three mechanisms of blockage repeat. Our treatment choices are similar, too. Again, all these therapies come late in the game. Prevention is the key as stroke recovery is difficult. The same diet considerations are recommended as for heart attack. Today, with a stroke, rapid assessment by a physician can reduce the severity or likelihood of a second one.

Cancer is, of course, the number two killer in North America. A diet as recommended for heart and stroke is an excellent start towards cancer prevention. The high fiber of many different fruits, vegetables, grains, and legumes will enhance your intake of protective phytochemicals. This includes lycopenes, anthocyanins, carotenoids, lutein, phytoestrogens, and flavonoids.

Digestive Disorders

Constipation can be the result of drug use or specific foods, but the vast majority of cases of constipation are the result of a diet low in fiber. If you suspect that low fiber is the reason you are constipated, increase fiber consumption slowly. You could also consider taking fiber supplement products like psyllium husk powder or some other lower bowel formula. Overuse of these types of products or sudden increase in fiber, however, will result in diarrhea. If diarrhea happens, make sure to drink lots of water to counteract dehydration. If diarrhea or abdominal pain persist, have it assessed by a clinician.

A good recommendation for fiber supplementation is 1-2 tablespoons of psyllium husk powder or 1-2 tablespoons natural bran or 1-2 tablespoons of ground flax daily. Increase fiber slowly to reduce the amount of gas.

Diarrhea (loose, watery stools) can be caused by food the body cannot tolerate, spoiled or rancid food, bacteria or viruses in food or water, caffeine, abuse of laxatives, parasites, and certain drugs. Chronic diarrhea accompanied by blood in the stool and fever may be a sign of infection.

No matter what the cause of your diarrhea, make sure you drink lots of water to prevent dehydration. Avoid foods that could make your diarrhea worse, like coffee, dairy products, spicy foods, and foods high in fat. A mild diarrhea can be allowed to run its course. It is the body's way of ridding itself of toxins. If it persists more than two weeks, see your health practitioner.

Gas and **Bloating** – As you've seen in the chapter on digestion, one of the reasons gas and bloating occur is as a result of your eating something that sits in the large bowel and ferments there (due to *indigestion*). Another reason it occurs is because you have eaten food that the stomach finds difficult to digest for whatever reason. Possibly your stomach is low on hydrochloric acid. This is quite likely if you are taking antacids or the H2 receptor medications which are marked by decreases in stomach acid. If you are experiencing emotional upset, this disturbs the "nervous" mechanism that controls stomach contraction and therefore proper food digestion. Some of the ways to prevent gas and bloating are:

- eat slowly and chew your food very well; there are digestive juices in your mouth, and the more you increase the surface area of your food by mulching it really well with your teeth, the less work your stomach and small intestine have to do;

- if you have a terrible problem with certain foods, avoid those foods or eat them in small quantities (cabbage, cruciferous vegetables such as cauliflower and Brussels sprouts, beans and peas, grapes and raisins);
- if you have been on a diet traditionally low in fiber, increase fiber intake slowly. A sudden increase in dietary fiber can cause severe cramps, gas, and bloating;
- look into several excellent digestive enzyme products available at your health food store to aid your stomach in digesting difficult foods;
- stay away from coffee, chocolate, wheat, dairy, soy, and other of the so-called "new foods" that may cause an allergic response in the body;
- eat only when you're hungry and stop when you're full;
- take two tablespoons of apple cider vinegar (the raw kind you buy in opaque bottles at your health food store) in half a glass of tepid water every morning on an empty stomach.[8] This restores the hydrochloric acid balance in the stomach, which decreases with age. When HCl is low, other enzymes for food digestion don't work as well either;
- don't talk incessantly while you're eating—you'll swallow a lot of air; and
- try to consume no water or any other liquids with your meal—you will dilute the stomach's digestive juices and make them less effective.

Irritable Bowel Syndrome is more than normal *motility* of large and small intestines. Typically associated with emotional stress, it is more likely the result of a food allergy. People with irritable bowel syndrome (IBS) experience diarrhea and pain—the latter resolves with a bowel movement.

Other names for IBS include *spastic colon* and *mucuous colitis*. The best solution is to first rule out the gastrointestinal disorders and then to increase fiber in the diet. Also, careful evaluation of allergies, as discussed in "Leaky Gut Syndrome" is useful.

Dr. Bill Code:
  My irritable bowel syndrome of many years resolved when I gave up wheat, dairy, and orange juice, i.e., my food allergies.

Gastrointestinal Disorders

Celiac Disease and **Tropical Sprue** are chronic intestinal malabsorption disorders caused by intolerance to the protein gluten, commonly found in wheat, rye, oats, and barley. (Breastfeeding helps to prevent the development of these diseases in infants and children.) Tropical sprue is like celiac and is triggered by a tropical illness (parasitic or bacterial, we don't know for sure). Sprue can often be resolved with a course of antibiotics. This course may require up to six months if the person continues to live in the tropics.

Diverticulitis occurs when small *diverticuli*, or pouch-like sacs are formed as a result of not enough fiber. Then, secondary constipation results in straining, high pressure in the large bowel, and these small outpouchings (like tiny balloons) on the wall. The diverticuli themselves are not painful, but if particles become lodged in them, they can cause pain, fever, and secondary infection. Antibiotics and/or emergency surgery may not be enough. Your best bet: increase fiber and *prevent* diverticulitis.

Heartburn *(reflux esophagitis)* is a burning sensation in the stomach and chest. It occurs when stomach acid backs up into the esophagus. This acid is very strong, and so irritates sensitive tissues. Normally, the flap of tissue at the bottom of the esophagus prevents hydrochloric acid from travelling upward out of the stomach. When, for whatever reason, this flap of tissue is compromised, the result is called *esophageal reflux disease*. There are a number of foods which can make heartburn or reflux disease worse, such as coffee, fatty or fried foods, citrus fruits, and alcohol. Ulcers or gallbladder problems can also make heartburn worse.

Hemorroids are enlarged veins in the lower rectum or anus. Hemorroids can be very painful and occasionally bleed. Emu oil can provide short-term relief when applied. Increased fiber will reduce constipation and hard, dry bowel movements. Many hemorroids resolve if people give up coffee (even decaffeinated). Surgery is hopefully avoided by the above.

Inflammatory Bowel Diseases – Crohn's disease and ulcerative colitis are inflammatory bowel diseases. Crohn's, or regional enteritis, usually involves the small intestine. Ulcerative colitis primarily involves the colon (large bowel). Both of these illnesses are autoimmune in origin. However, the initiating features are unknown. Canada has the highest incidence of inflammatory bowel disease in the world. It is possible a lack of vitamin D and high intake of wheat are factors in their prevalence.

Leaky Gut Syndrome
Leaky gut could well be the initial step in many of our chronic ailments—especially autoimmune disorders. Gut (gastrointestinal) troubles are one of the most common reasons for physicians to send you to a specialist. Your health care practitioner may use the term "irritable bowel syndrome".

Dr. Bill Code:
> I was handed that label in my mid-thirties. My complaints were abdominal cramps, intermittent gas, constipation or loose, runny bowel movements, and the

ultimate challenge—"occasional fatigue". Migraine headaches occurred every 1-2 weeks—especially if a Chinook (strong west winds bringing sudden and dramatic changes in atmospheric pressure) blew in from the Rockies. We lived in Calgary at that time. The only symptoms of leaky gut that I didn't have was aching joints! Physical exams revealed tenderness in part of the abdomen on deep palpitation (pushing down of physician's hand). Lab tests showed normal blood count and no nasty bacteria or parasites on stool culture.[7]

Leaky gut is your intestines acting as a porous or too-open sieve of foods into your bloodstream. These "too large" food particles travel to your liver and in most cases continue on into your bloodstream. These "chunks" include the regular digested fare of simple sugars, fatty acids, amino acids, and peptides (two or three amino acids together). In addition, these "chunks" include bacteria, fungi, parasites, undigested proteins, fat, and other particles which would usually not be absorbed.

Now, our immune system is our brave defender so it attacks these foreign invaders. If it does this, it will eliminate the foreign proteins. However, our body has self-proteins with their own markers on them. What could happen? Yes, our immune system could attack one of our own group of cells because it looks so much like a foreign protein. The result is autoimmune disease, i.e., our body attacking a part of itself. For example, if the foreign protein looks like the lining cells of a joint (synovium), we now have rheumatoid arthritis. Similar examples include SLE (lupus), multiple sclerosis, thyroiditis (low or hypothyroid result), diabetes, regional enteritis (Crohn's disease), ulcerative colitis, and Raynaud's disease (a blood vessel inflammation).

How can we reverse this autoimmune disease? We have at least two choices. We can dampen or suppress our immune system (e.g., cortisone, methotrexate, NSAIDs). Another option is to "heal" the leaky gut. How? By removing the drug, food, or infection that triggered the leaky gut in the first place. This means stopping the cortisone, NSAIDs, or broad spectrum antibiotics. Other choices would be treating the parasite or bacteria that started "leaking". Finally, and perhaps most commonly, is removing the food which our gut and body is now sensitized or allergic to.

Dr. Bill Code:

Detecting which food is the trigger can be easy, but may be difficult. I discovered that wheat and wheat products started my migraine headaches. When I gave up wheat, my headaches became rare. Also, many of my bowel complaints stopped if I avoided wheat, milk, and oranges. Could these be a factor in my multiple sclerosis? I believe they are. Recently, I broke both wheat (lasagne) and milk (ice cream) diet rules. The result was a headache and the worse fatigue in weeks. For folks without obvious signals of what foods they are allergic to, I suggest: (a) elimination diets (by a qualified dietician); (b) electrodermal allergy testing; or (c) ELISA – an expensive blood test.

First you must find a qualified health care professional to help you on this road.

Ulcers occur in the stomach and duodenum when the lining of the stomach fails to protect the stomach itself from digestive juices. The stomach, in effect, begins to digest itself. An ulcer is sometimes caused by an excess of stomach acid, and sometimes by lower than required amounts of protective mucus. Sometimes both conditions exist. *Peptic (stomach) ulcers* affect about 10 per cent of the population, and are closely related to stress, since stress elevates the production of acid. Follow our recommendations for diet and good health in this book and ulcers should improve. The bacteria *Heliobacter pylori* is linked to stomach ulcers. This type of ulcer is best treated by antibiotics under the care of a physician.

CHAPTER 4

Weight Loss for Longevity and Vibrant Health

D o you want to lose weight? Have you been struggling with weight problems most of your life? Does it seem like no matter what you do, you can't seem to shed those unwanted pounds?

If so, you are not alone. Billions of dollars are spent in the U.S. and Canada every year on weight loss products ranging from memberships in fitness clubs to special shakes to "diet" pills. On television, commercials promise miraculous weight loss. News programs discuss weight loss advances while doctors caution (at the tail end of these newscasts) that, "Still, the best way to lose weight is to eat sensibly and exercise."

So, what's the problem? How many years have we heard this advice? The problem is multi-faceted, but it takes tackling only *two* simple concepts that will make weight loss possible for most of you. Just two. If you can get your head around these two vital truths, you will be miles ahead of other people.

The first truth: *most food manufacturers have only the profits of their companies at heart.* If this were not true, they wouldn't manufacture food loaded with trans fats, sugar and chemical preservatives, additives, and colors. It is these foods which are making us fat and unhealthy. Not only that, but their aggressive marketing tactics leave our brains—and our ability to discern and think for ourselves—exhausted. The next time you are at an intersection in suburban North America, look around. What do you see? Fast food of every description—donuts, pizza, burgers, and on and on and on. While most of us may enjoy a fast food burger *very occasionally*, for many people, this food is their staple diet. This is alarming, but unfortunately true. It is the ingredients in these "foods" that are making us all sick.

But that's not all. If you walk down the aisle at your grocery store, you will see that *everything* you were once able to only buy as a whole food (for example, the humble potato, fish, cheese, apples) is now also available in a chopped up, mashed up, chemical-laden, trans fat laden, colorized, processed, *manufactured* version of the original. The new packaged "food" bears little resemblance to the original—not in taste and certainly not in nutritional quality. A sandwich isn't a sandwich unless you've loaded it with mayonnaise. Pasta isn't pasta until you've drowned it in fat-laden Alfredo sauce. Salad isn't salad unless you've poured on bottled salad dressing designed to harden even the hardiest arteries.

Most people, when searching for a snack at home, rarely consider *whole foods* as snack items. In this regard, it is possible that some of us are getting better. We are now grabbing apples, a handful of cherries, a banana, or an orange more readily than we did some years ago. But a snack seems more like a snack when it's high fat (donuts or muffins) or comes out of a box or bag: cookies or potato chips (both also high in fat); if we are thirsty, we dig around in the refrigerator for a can of pop.

Where and when did this turnaround in our thinking occur? *How* did it occur? Again, we owe it all to marketing. The next time you are watching TV at dinner time or late at night, count the percentage of commercials that advertise snack food—pizza (frozen and take out), chocolate bars, corn chips, sugary pops. When you watch the advertising carefully, you will see that

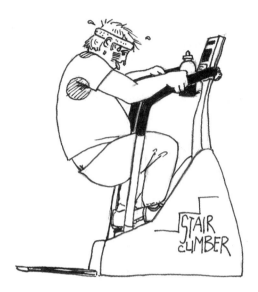

besides being promised thirst quenching or growl satisfying fare, we are also going to mountain bike more professionally, hit a better golf ball, swing a more eloquent tennis racquet, get that date, or have *a lot* of fun in an elevator.

Be suspicious of foods that promise to deliver health, but actually deliver little more than sugar and water. Many "juices" are really only colored water and several varieties of sugar with a few drops of juice added. In some cases, the word "drink" or "punch" on the packaging will tip you off.

Worse yet are beer commercials. Since when do people who appear in beer commercials look like the people who hang out in bars? They never do. People who hang out in bars have beer guts and pasty, grey complexions. If they don't actively smoke, they do so passively, and their outward appearance certainly shows this. Beer commercials promise love, popularity, wide expanses of beaches, or wild, hilarious parties with no consequences. We won't attempt to discuss the morality of drinking beer or any other alcohol. However, consuming alcohol to excess—and it's anybody's guess where that line is—is an activity that is best avoided. After all, there are often adverse circumstances beer advertisers will of course not warn us about.[1] Besides, alcohol is high in calories and sugar and devoid of any nutrition.

If we can block out this negative advertising, we will, as I said, be miles ahead of most people. Another positive benefit to learning how to do this—besides being good for the waistline—is that it removes guilt, tension, and temptation. If you don't eat that kind of food, then you don't eat that kind of food. Period. You can't be tempted because it's off your list. This is surprisingly easy once you are fully there, once you are fully committed to the concept. It is a much more peaceful way to live, rather than knowing how bad it is for you, telling yourself you really shouldn't, and then eating it anyway, feeling guilty afterwards. Suddenly, it seems like it makes sense (not only nutritionally but also financially) to stop in at the food store next to the burger place and pick up a bag of apples. Surely apples are also food? A couple will hold you until you get home.

This is not rocket science. Once you understand what this food is doing to your body, and once you start to comprehend how you've been a pawn in the game of their ever-increasing profits, it is not hard to shun some foods for good. You also begin to see just how hard it is to get a nutritious meal on the go. As a matter of fact, it's virtually impossible. The answer is to cook for yourself (remember I told you it would be simple, but not necessarily easy), and when you don't have time to cook or prepare take-along food, eat whole food. Since when was a carrot (organic, please, if at all possible—that goes for all your foods) or an apple not a food? Why does it have to be handed to you from a take-out window or munched from a bag purchased at the gas station to be appealing and qualify as food?

The answer is that we have been so brainwashed with advertising, that we feel we are somehow "missing something" by avoiding this food. We are missing the love, fun, adventure, better golf swing, or whatever, that clever marketing and advertising tactics have convinced us we will get, if we only eat their food, or drink their drink.

Be an original! Don't fall sway to this relentless marketing. Think of it as water torture. Drip by agonizing drip, you slowly give up the right to make up your own mind about what's right for you to take into your body. *Make up your own mind,* based on the information you receive here, and any other *non-fad* health reading you may do (please see our bibliography for suggested further reading).

Weight loss or weight maintenance ought to be closely tied to health anyway. Would you eat burgers, chips, and chocolate bars if they didn't cause weight gain but were still unhealthy for you? Probably. Would you eat something you'd never seen before just because a commercial on TV told you it was okay and/or cool to eat it? Possibly.

The point here is that there is food and then there is *non-food.* Anything altered drastically from its original state (*processed* cheese, potato *chips,* etc.) is a non-food. The list could go on endlessly, but let us take you through a walk of some of the more common items in most people's grocery carts: white bread, white pasta, bagels, fish sticks, TV dinners, fruit cocktail, salad dressings and mayonnaises, cereal (we could write a whole *chapter* on cereal), toaster pastries, specialty coffees, juice *cocktails,* ice cream, bacon, frozen pizza, sausages, corn chips, salsa, deli pasta or potato salads, puddings, cake & muffin mixes, and imitation pancake syrup.

Of course, speaking of cereal, advertisers tend to be rather unscrupulous when marketing to children. One advertiser actually shows children flicking broccoli off their plates at dinner time or feeding it to the dog because it's "yucky." How this will ever instill good eating habits in our children is anybody's guess. Another (and broccoli seems to be a favourite to pick on) has a friend staying over for dinner because mom is putting a cheese sauce on the broccoli—apparently the only possible way it can be stomached. The cheese sauce is *processed* cheese. What percentage of processed cheese can honestly be said to be good for you? And why isn't broccoli okay on its own?

Claudia Tiefisher:

> North Americans have developed a cereal culture. I remember when I was a child standing in front of the cereal aisle for what must have seemed like hours to my parents, deciding which one I wanted this week. I was usually swayed by the cartoons on the box, the commercials I'd seen on TV, or the toy I knew I'd find inside. Growing up in Canada, even Wonder Bread® was a source of wonder and amazement to me. It was so desirable because you couldn't buy it in Canada—it was only available in the U.S. On one shopping trip I begged for some Wonder Bread, thinking I'd be as happy as the kids I'd seen on TV when *they* were eating *their* Wonder Bread sandwiches. I distinctly remember being disappointed that it was, after all, just fluffy, not especially special, ordinary white bread.

Other children's manufacturers try to make fruit fun with fruit "leather" that can be stretched, bent, and twisted into "fun" shapes before it's eaten. Our feeling is that it would be better to teach a child to appreciate fruit in its natural form, not in some altered form that has had sugar, chemicals, and preservatives added to it and cartoons painted on the box that the product comes in. Dollar-wise, the food value is in a bag of apples instead of a box of fruit leather.

All this stuff gets in our heads and makes decisions for us as we walk down the supermarket aisle. Resist it and you will lose weight. Buy whole foods, prepare them yourself, and you will lose weight. Guaranteed.

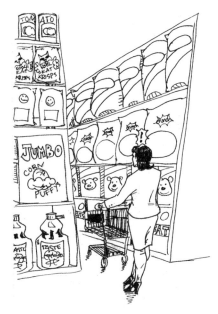

Now for the second truth: *You will not lose weight by starving yourself, living off bagels, and swearing off fat.* Ah, yes. Life used to be simple, didn't it? There was an easy "truism" that made so much sense 20 or 30 years ago. Restrict calories and you would lose weight. While this is, strictly speaking, true, many people went about it the wrong way, eliminating the wrong types of foods and not paying any attention to *what their bodies needed to function.* We'll get more into why this is true in a moment.

There are other reasons why this starve-yourself approach doesn't work. When you restrict calories to an excessive degree, you signal your body that there's a shortage of food. You have to remember that we have been evolving for a very short period of time, physiologically speaking—a blink of an eye, really. Our cave-dwelling ancestors lived on very, very lean protein (wild meat is much leaner than the meat animals raised on today's farms), and *gathered* grains, vegetables, fruits, nuts, seeds, and berries. *Gathered* means nothing was cultivated, and so there was never an abundant supply of any type of food. This gathered food was sparse, so the calories obtained from it likely made up a small percentage of the diet. The meat was lean, but it was also our primary source of fat. Hence, we obtained *protein*—necessary for tissue-building, repair, growth, and also providing food energy—from meat. We also obtained *fat*—which was, besides protein, the most desirable type of food we could get, as it was rich in calories, much harder to come by than carbohydrates, and would stay with us for a long time after being consumed. *Protein* and *fat* were the two things we were after all those years ago. Of course, back then we didn't know the differences between fat, carbohydrates, and protein, from a scientific point of view. We only knew what satisifed us and what we had cravings for.

But before you go thinking you can start living off T-bone steaks, think again. Our ancestors also received their fat from other sources such as leafy vegetables, seeds, and nuts. The meat they ate, as mentioned earlier, was lean; the meat we have today is much fattier. The other types of fat provided them with *essential fatty acids*—you know all about those now.

Eat lean meats and remove the fat. Birds' meat does not marble the way beef, pork, venison, and lamb do. If you remove visible fat and skin from poultry, you will avoid most of the fat. Consider emu, ostrich, chicken, and turkey—the more natural the better.

Of course, our cave-dwelling ancestors had other health advantages we cannot possibly hope to duplicate these days. They relied on manual labour for everything, had clean food sources and a pristine environment. Another note of interest: before fire was discovered, all food must have been eaten raw. Therefore, beans and legumes were not consumed as part of this diet because they couldn't be consumed raw. While beans and legumes are an excellent source of fiber, complex carbohydrates, and protein (and are devoid of damaging fats), they are hard to digest. If you have irritable bowel syndrome or some other lower bowel digestive complaint, it may be advisable to limit consumption of these foods or eliminate them from your diet altogether. After all, they have not been part of the natural human diet for very long at all.

Back then, there was much celebration when a large kill was made—there would be food for all and the food energy stayed with them for days and days. But, in the more numerous and lengthy stretches of subsisting on berries and nuts, the body compensated by slowing *metabolism.* No food coming signalled imminent starvation and the need to conserve the food energy—both temporarily stored (as glycogen) and more permanently stored (as fat). What this means in practical terms is that if you normally consume a varied diet consisting of 3,000 calories a day, your body will operate at a certain level, like a furnace that is fed so much coal. If you suddenly drop that to 1,000 calories a day, a number of things will happen. The first thing is your body responds by drastically slowing metabolism. It thinks you're not going to have another kill for many days, maybe even a week or two. In response, it needs to conserve what fuel it has. So, if you normally burn 200 calories an hour crossing the African Savannah, your body is now efficiently burning only about 75 calories per hour (these are hypothetical numbers simply meant to illustrate how your body responds). *The same thing happens when you starve yourself today.* Our bodies have not evolved much at all since those days, and yet our diets have been drastically altered.

The second thing that happens is *you deprive your body of the nutrition that it needs to function.* When you feel sluggish and low on energy, or if your immune system is not up to par, it means you are not getting the nutrition you need. You may be compounding the problem by compromising your health in some other way, like not getting enough rest, experiencing too much stress, smoking, or drinking too much alcohol. But let's focus on the nutrition. What is so hard for most people to grasp (but which you should have a clear understanding of now), is the importance of essential fatty acids in your diet. Without these fatty acids, you body cannot function properly. You end up with foggy thinking, poor energy transfer in your cells, and a tendency to weight gain. As we've said before, the first, biggest, and most common mistake people make when attempting to lose weight is they cut as much fat as possible from their diet. *You will not lose weight by doing this.* You may lose weight at first, but once you start eating "normally" again, you will quickly regain the lost weight. Worse, your body will continue to respond to the starvation by adding even *more fat* as storage, thinking that, eventually, it will encounter another lean time such as the one it has just suffered through. It is acting in self-defense.

The other reason you will not lose weight like this is because your liver, which is the main fat-burning engine of your body, is damaged for two reasons—an excess of toxins and an excess of bad fat. Unless you clean up your liver, you can expect a body that is functioning below optimal to continue to do so. This requires a program of strict adherence to foods that are *liver friendly* and a swearing-off of foods that are *liver toxic*. A complete list of these foods is provided later in this chapter. Once you clean up your liver, your body can properly metabolize fats again and weight loss follows naturally.

Your body cannot function without essential fatty acids (see Chapters 1 and 2). Think of essential fatty acids as nature's "diet" pill. No, EFAs are not a cure-all, but without them, lasting, healthy weight loss is next to impossible. Of course, there are other, equally important nutritional components like the right amount of calories, good proteins, paying attention to possible food allergies, vitamins, minerals, fiber, and water. The problem with the essential fatty acids, the reason we single them out as often and as prominently as we do, is this: *because we have been taught that fats make us fat, because we avoid fats at all costs, because we cut fats from our diets in an attempt to lose weight, and because essential fatty acids—in their correct form—are not easy to get in the standard North American diet, we must almost treat them like medicine.*

Getting essential fatty acids into your diet is not difficult. Once you know what foods contain them, you can start incorporating these foods into your family's daily routine. But you will also see how not knowing enough about them can lead to essential fatty acid deficiencies, now considered to be reaching epidemic proportions in the North American population. *Do whatever it takes to get these EFAs into your diet. The balance of the omega-3 and omega-6 fatty acids should be a 1:6 ratio.*

At the same time, it is important to cut down on *bad fats*. We've talked about this at length in the chapter on fats, but it bears mentioning again here. You should limit your intake of saturated fats (those present in most animal products) and eliminate your intake of *trans* fats. Do this correctly, and rest assured, weight loss will follow.

We told you that the second truth was that living off bagels won't help you lose weight. This was all the rage a few years ago. High carbohydrate, low fat diets were seen as the solution to people's weight problems. We've talked, too, about the fact that even though we are cutting all this fat from our diets, we are heavier, on average, than we were 20 years ago. The reason for this is twofold. One has been explained at length in this book— we aren't getting the right fats, and we aren't getting enough essential fatty acids. The other reason is that when we eat carbohydrates, especially refined carbohydrates that contain little or no fiber (like white bagels), the sugars are quickly broken down for use by the body. This would be good except for one thing: there is too much sugar present for the body to use right then and there. Because the food lacks fiber, digestion happens quickly (remember how fiber acts like the brakes on the uptake of sugar into the bloodstream). Whatever the bloodstream can't absorb for instant energy is converted into glycogen. The hor-

mone responsible for this conversion is insulin, which is manufactured by the pancreas. Some glycogen is sent for storage in
the muscles, and if there is still some blood sugar left over, the
body will continue to secrete more and more insulin, packing up
the overload of carbohydrates for transport to the fat deposit
centres of the body. The more insulin is made, the more sugar
will be shipped off for storage as fat, since the bloodstream can
only absorb so much for use as active energy.

When we haven't eaten for a long time, our pancreas responds by stimulating the liver to release stored glycogen (glycogen is the stored form of glucose). The hormone responsible for
this is glucagon. This process keeps our blood sugar (i.e., the
amount of glucose in the blood) from dipping dangerously low.
Without sugar in our blood, our brains would quickly shut
down and we would go into shock or a coma. Extensive "starvation" of the brain of glucose leads, ultimately, to death.

Ups and downs of blood glucose are what diabetics suffer
from. A person with diabetes must be very diligent about maintaining as stable a blood sugar level as possible. The way to do
this, of course, is to restrict simple sugars like alcohol, candy,
and fruit juices. But there are a host of other simple sugars
(termed *simple carbohydrates* because they lack fiber and are constructed mainly of *monosaccharides*) which are to be equally
avoided. These include mashed potatoes, white flour pasta,
white bagels, breads and pastries, cookies and cakes, even a teaspoon of sugar in tea (though diabetics can consume some sugar
in controlled amounts).

In Type I (insulin-dependent) diabetes, the body makes virtually no insulin. Consequently, eating simple sugars without
accompanying insulin injections leaves the body unable to process the sugar. In other words, there is no process whereby the
sugar is converted into a form that can be stored by the body.
Therefore, all the sugar consumed would surge directly into the
bloodstream. Type II (non-insulin dependent) diabetes is char-

acterized by the presence of insulin, but the body is insulin-resistant. This type of diabetes can often be controlled without insulin injections by adherence to a good diet, maintaining correct body weight, and by exercise. Insulin partially regulates the metabolism of fats and proteins as well.

The problem with the so-called "high carbohydrate, low fat" diets is twofold. The first problem is that they didn't tell us *high carbohydrate* actually meant high *complex* carbohydrate. This means foods like raw vegetables and fruit (that contain the fiber when you eat them, i.e., as opposed to the juices of vegetables and fruits). If you only consume carbohydrates devoid of any fiber, your body responds by making too much insulin and you have the problem described above.

The second problem is that they told us low fat. But we are now seeing that low fat diets are not the answer to weight loss, as we've tried to explain at some length. Not only did they err in telling us to eat low fat (we need some fat—saturated, polyunsaturated, and monounsaturated, and also cholesterol), but … and here it comes again … *we need those essential fatty acids.* Did any of the authors of these books make that clear enough? That low fat didn't mean restricting *all* fats? Did they warn us that low fat would lead to poor energy transfer between cells, poor liver function, poor nerve function, and lower levels of energy in general? Did they mention that it is the essential fatty acids that are primarily responsible for the body's ability to manufacture cell walls, enzymes, and hormones—*vitally* important to the good health of our bodies, as we've seen in the insulin/glucagon examples above? *This* is where these diets have fallen down.

We offer you a *new* way of thinking about what you eat.

First of all, *food is not the enemy.* We need food, and who wouldn't agree that a well-prepared meal, full of color and aroma, is one of life's greatest pleasures? Make food your friend again. Thoroughly acquaint yourself with what's good for you, what isn't, what's vital, and what's okay to have once in a while, and it will become a part of you. Remember that it takes about 21 days to establish a new habit. Start eating this way now and in three weeks it will be routine. You should not feel deprived, knowing that you are giving your body the vital nutrition it needs for optimum health. And you shouldn't feel hungry, because you may eat as many of the health-friendly foods as you wish. You will find new ways to prepare old favourites. You will feel lighter, more energetic, your thinking will be clearer, and you will have a more positive attitude. Mild depressions will lift.

Before launching into the plan, there's just one more thing. Many of the weight loss problems we see today—besides being caused to a great degree by the misconceptions and misinformation we've already talked about—exist because so many of us have an underfunctioning, or *sluggish*, liver. The plan proposed in this book is meant to cleanse the liver and allow it to perform at its peak once again.

A Word About the Liver

The liver is an amazing organ. The body's heaviest, it also, arguably, has the most important job. It is amazing because the liver can be damaged or up to 75% of its weight removed and, under most circumstances, will regenerate. The liver's job is not only to neutralize any toxins you ingest with your food, but also those toxins that are inhaled or that are absorbed transdermally (through the skin). Your lungs and kidneys also process and neutralize toxins. That's why you must drink lots of water, never, ever smoke, and avoid second-hand smoke as much as possible.

Toxins you ingest include residual pesticides and herbicides on your food. They include preservatives, coloring, and artificial flavours. They include nitrites (present in most smoked foods, including bacon), substances meant to keep food from clumping (such as in instant hot chocolate), or separating (such as in mayonnaise or bottled salad dressings). They also include trans fats, as these are made up of fatty acid molecules (as explained in the chapter on fats) that the body perceives as being foreign (i.e., unnatural).

The liver is responsible for neutralizing all these toxins. When your liver is overloaded with work (think of your in-basket vs. your out-basket at work), your liver (the in-basket) gets bloated with fluids, toxins, and partially digested fats. Every drop of blood in your body goes through your liver every three to four minutes. And every drop of blood from your digestive system (i.e., from your small intestine) filters through your liver before going on to the rest of the body.

When the liver is overburdened, it is usually only for a short period of time. There is a short back-up (which you may feel as bloating, gas, or indigestion), but then everything gets rolling again and things go back to normal. Sometimes, however, over time, there can be a chronic build-up of fats and toxins accumulating in the liver, and it is this condition which causes so many of the overweight conditions we see today. Even worse, a sluggish liver creates a whole host of other symptoms:[2]

- circles under the eyes
- a coated tongue
- bad breath
- sluggish or foggy thinking
- mood swings
- constipation
- depression
- can exacerbate (make worse) or trigger allergic conditions
- headaches
- poor regulation of blood sugar
- bloated abdomen
- excessive body heat
- an inability to tolerate fatty foods
- can lead to gallbladder disease and gallstones
- chronic fatigue syndrome

The reason so many of these symptoms show up is that the whole body is overloaded with toxins because of the liver's inability to keep up. Though the liver is a real trooper and works hard even when it is overburdened, it sometimes, in effect, throws up its hands because it has gone beyond the point of being able to cope. It then dumps toxins, partly digested proteins, and semi-digested fats directly into your bloodstream and bile without these substances first being neutralized or converted into a form your body can use. This can cause big trouble, as now you are forcing your immune system to take over. The immune system is also amazing in how it handles toxic overload, but if you force it into overdrive too often, the result can be autoimmunity. Here's how this works.

If a partly digested protein that your body has a sensitivity to sneaks past your liver and goes directly into your bloodstream, your immune response is to find the foreign invader (it doesn't recognize it in its present form) and destroy it. This immune response sends white blood cells to the site (this could be one single spot on the body or all over if the foreign invader has travelled through your bloodstream). This is important. When you have an injury (say you cut yourself), these cells are vital to help prevent infection. Internally, the cells working to destroy the invader give off heat and oxygen—sort of like their exhaust system. This "heat" results in inflammation, so to speak. When it is in one spot (such as in rheumatoid arthritis where the body attacks joint tissue), the result is redness, swelling, heat, and loss of use. When it is all over, the result is achiness, tender muscles, swollen lymph nodes, or possibly chronic fatigue syndrome or fibromyalgia.

If the white blood cell immune "troops" are successful in destroying the invader, life goes on. However, sometimes, especially in the case of proteins, these immune molecules or cells decide one of our own self-proteins looks like a foreign protein. Now our immune troops go after that protein or cell type from our own body. Your body is now going after itself—after its own, healthy tissues—creating what is called an "autoimmune" condition. You read about autoimmune conditions in the last chapter. Now you understand, in a very basic way, how this occurs.

For instance, in multiple sclerosis, the theory is that the body begins to attack the myelin sheath—the protective fatty covering that surrounds our nerve cells. This results in a misfiring or lack of communication between those nerve cells. In osteoarthritis, the body attacks the cartilage between certain bones and also the synovial fluid there, which attracts and holds water, vital to the cushioning of those joints. It is now speculated that even cancer has components of autoimmune disease.

Facilitate the clean-up of the liver; allow it to function optimally once again, and you will start to metabolize fats correctly, leading to natural weight loss and super high-quality, high-energy health. This is the foundation upon which this eating program rests. If you feel your liver is quite weak, or you have suffered extreme liver damage such as hepatitis, cirrhosis, or removal of a portion of your liver due to injury, you should take a liver cleansing supplement or a collection of herbs to help facilitate the healing process.[3]

Liver-friendly foods
(where it applies, try to get organic whenever possible)
Raw & dried fruit
Raw vegetables
Whole-grain breads and other high fiber foods
Raw nuts & seeds
Cold pressed virgin vegetable & seed oils
Legumes (beans, peas, & lentils)
Hummus, tahini and nut spreads from the health food store
Oily, fresh, cold-water sea foods such as tuna, salmon, sardines, & mackerel

Liver-toxic foods
Trans fats
Excessive saturated fats
More than four alcoholic drinks weekly; Tobacco
Raw fish
Smoked or deep-fried food of any kind

If you have chronic digestive complaints or allergy problems, try eliminating dairy foods from your diet. If you are trying to lose weight and return your liver to optimum function, eliminate all liver-toxic foods while you are on the liver cleanse diet. Coffee should always be limited to two cups daily. More than that wreaks havoc with your nervous system, leaving you in a perpetual cycle of nervous energy and exhaustion.

This program can be followed for eight weeks or for much longer. There is enough nutrition—if you eat a variety of the liver-friendly foods outlined above—to survive and thrive in excellent health. Some people stay on this program for the rest of their lives, having once tried it, simply because they've never felt better. Buy a few high quality vegetarian, vegan cookbooks. You should restrict your intake of red meats while you are healing your liver and losing weight. However, meat is an excellent source of many vital nutrients and if you decide to eat it (as opposed to going vegetarian), make sure you know where the meat comes from. Insist on organic or natural meat that has not been injected with hormones or antibiotics. To a large degree, it is these chemicals which have overburdened our livers, resulting in weight gain and poor health—not just the fat present in the meats. Eat only lean cuts (remember our discussion about fatty meats earlier in this chapter). On the program, you may eat organic chicken or other types of birds like emu, ostrich, or turkey, and organic, free-range eggs. If you elect to follow the program for life, you may certainly introduce red meats. Just remember to know where they come from and pick the leanest cuts.

The Eight-Week Program

1. About forty per cent of your diet should consist of raw fruits and vegetables. These foods contain natural antibiotics, digestive enzymes, chlorophyll, roughage, carotenoids, bioflavonoids, and other healthy substances that will help heal your liver and cleanse your bowel.

2. If the food you eat is nutrient deficient, you can expect to remain hungry until you get sufficient nutrients. For this reason, if you wish to remain slim, you should eat foods that are high in nutrition. Also, make sure foods are high in fiber—food passes through the digestive tract much smoother if it is high in fiber.

3. A top quality liver cleansing formula should contain substances that are known to feed and to cleanse the liver. Dandelion (*Taxicum officinalis*) has been used to cleanse the liver in traditional herbal medicine for centuries. *Citrus aurantium* has thermogenic capabilities. This means that it burns off extra calories and therefore fat. Milk thistle (*Silybum marianum*) is possibly the best herb available for detoxification and protection of the liver. *Garcinia cambogia* helps to increase the amount of fat burned as fuel, helps to reduce the amount of fat produced and stored in adipose tissue, and helps to suppress the appetite.

4. Beef, lamb, pork, venison, and dairy products, as you know, are high in saturated fatty acids. While these have received a bad rap over the years (worse than they deserve), a damaged liver has a hard time metabolizing them, and therefore they contribute to weight gain and to an inability to lose weight. There should be no more than four servings of this group of foods per week during the liver cleansing program. If you must eat dairy foods, opt for lower-fat dairy foods during the cleanse.

5. Damaged fats are fats that have suffered high heat and/or high pressure. In order to make fats more spreadable,

manufacturers take liquid oils such as canola or corn and damage them with high heat, high pressure, or hydrogenation. Examples of this are margarine, shortening, and spreadable cheese. Frying fats will also damage them. Avoid all deep-fried foods at all times, not just when on the liver cleanse program. Also, avoid hydrogenated and partially hydrogenated vegetable oil products.

Pointers on helping to maintain a healthy liver during the liver cleanse program:

- Probably the single most important thing you will do is to completely avoid liver toxic foods. This is vital. No matter how much liver friendly and liver supporting foods and supplements you consume, your liver will function sub-optimally if you continue to feed it what it considers poisons.
- You don't have to count calories. If you listen to your body, you will take your cues correctly. Don't listen to fast or convenience food manufacturers (nacho corn chips won't make your life more fun, no matter how the commercials try to convince you). *Listen to your body.* If you're not hungry at mealtime (and you may find your appetite decreasing), have just a small salad with some flax oil sprinkled on top. It's important to eat only when you're hungry and to stop when you're full. Don't stuff yourself because something tastes good. You may be satisfying a psychological urge, but consider what you are doing to your body.
- It only takes 15 to 20 minutes before you start to feel satisfied. Notice *satisfied* as opposed to *full*. By the time you are feeling full, you have probably already overeaten. Stop when you are no longer hungry.
- Avoid foods containing artificial chemicals such as flavouring, coloring, artificial sweeteners, and preservatives. Where possible, try to eat organically grown food.
- Chew foods slowly and thoroughly in order to ensure com-

plete digestion. This means having healthy teeth! Brush twice daily and floss once daily. See your dentist twice a year. Healthy teeth can take 6 years off your "real" age.

- Drink at least eight glasses of pure or filtered water daily.
- Avoid processed meats and fast foods.
- Cut down on sugar intake and absolutely avoid artificial sweeteners.
- Avoid foods that have caused bloating or otherwise upset you in the past. If you must eat them, it may be wise to take a digestive enzyme.
- Eat bread only if it is the high fiber variety and free of artificial chemicals.
- Substitute products such as avocado, tahini, and hummus for the usual butter on your bread.
- Avoid dairy products, especially the full fat variety.
- First thing upon rising, take two tablespoons of apple cider vinegar in a half glass of tepid water. This helps to restore the acid balance in your stomach and will aid in digestion. Make sure you get the organic kind from the health food store. It should be raw, unfiltered, and unprocessed and bottled in opaque, brown bottles.
- Following the apple cider vinegar, drink a glass of freshly squeezed orange or orange/grapefruit juice. This will give you vitamin C and lots of other nutrients. If you find straight juice too acidic, dilute it half and half with water.
- At some point in the day, have a glass of carrot/celery/parsley juice. Make sure you are using organic fruits and vegetables, if at all possible. Carrots, celery, and parsley are known for their liver cleansing qualities. Beets are also very efficient at cleansing the liver.
- Eat raw fruits and vegetables throughout the day. To avoid excess sugar, eat more vegetables than fruit.
- In order to get sufficient essential fatty acids, it is necessary to eat fats. But, avoid damaged fats and excessive saturated

fats. Ground flax seeds (see Chapter 6) will help this.
- Do not eat when under emotional stress.
- Minimize your meat intake. You can get protein by combining three of these four foods at a meal: legumes, nuts, seeds, and grains.
- Take your supplements as described in Chapter 6.

Claudia Tiefisher:
Please see the Appendix—*Testimonials* for my personal experience with this program.

During the liver cleanse, weight loss may not occur at all during a two to six-week period. During this time, the liver is cleansing. Don't lose heart. Expect weight loss to occur after the cleanse has taken place. For this reason, it is a good idea to *stay off the scale*. Instead, measure your success by how you feel and how your clothes fit. You can weigh yourself after the eight weeks or long after that.

Finally, remember that weight loss is for life, not just for the reunion dress you want desperately to be able to fit into. Quick and simple weight loss is never lasting and never healthy. You should lose no more than a few pounds a month. The more you incorporate lifetime healthy eating habits as you are on a weight loss regimen, the healthier you will feel, and the more energetic you will be. You stand a better chance of avoiding society's degenerative, autoimmune diseases. You will likely live longer.

Avoid trans fats, limit saturated fats, eat lots of fiber, drink lots of water, and *get your essential fatty acids*. The next chapter will give you a good primer for exercise—a crucial component of lasting weight loss and lasting good health.

CHAPTER 5

Exercise for Energy, Vibrant Health, and Longevity

As adults, we all struggle with finding the time, inclination, inspiration, motivation, and desire to exercise. Some people who exercise liken it to brushing their teeth—something which has to be done, every day, whether you like it or not. They set up treadmills in front of their TV sets and go for an hour or so a night.

Most of us live in the city and work at full-time jobs away from home. Most of you reading this probably have numerous duties that stretch your time in every direction, leaving you exhausted and with little time left over for yourself. Any way you can work physical activity into your daily life is a plus. If you live in an area where the climate is amenable, it might be best to take your exercise out of doors. Studies have shown that runners who run outdoors and concentrate on a spot on the horizon—that is, they keep their heads up and forward rather than watching their feet or the road in front of them—have better utilization of oxygen and can run farther and faster.

This is interesting, because it suggests that the psychological side of exercising plays a big role in the success of your venture. Know this: if you decide to start on a running program, you will probably have to drag yourself out of the house on many, many occasions for the first few weeks. This is normal. But do whatever it takes. Call it a "no option" rule for your life. You do it, no matter what.

There are many benefits to exercising. One of the keys to truly understanding the benefits, and to make exercise seem easier on the hard days, is recognizing that it is more than just a means to an end (a healthier, leaner, fitter body). Your body was meant to be used. Your muscles, bones, joints, and organs all benefit from movement. Your psyche, soul, and brain benefit from movement as well. Like any machine, your body will become rusty if you do not use it. Your muscles will atrophy (become limp and ineffectual) and whether you gain weight or not as a result of your inactivity, you put your organs and joints in danger. Why? Because if your muscles are toned and fit, you stand a far smaller chance of injury. You are less likely to trip and fall, less likely to reach for something only to have it result in a pulled muscle.

Being fit makes life more fun. You don't feel compelled to find excuses to not "join in" some activity—for whatever reason. Maybe you are uncomfortable about your body. Maybe you can't take part because you lack the strength or skills. Probably the reason most people don't participate in certain activities—a round of golf with friends, doubles tennis with the neighbours, or trying something new like water skiing—is because we give in to our fears. We fear we'll look stupid, and this is rooted in a low level of self-confidence. Confidence increases exponentially when a person exercises regularly. It is thrilling to huff and puff your way through a 20 minute walk, and six months later to be running several miles. The sense of accomplishment is extreme and the feeling of "I did it!" stays with you no matter what you endeavour to do in your daily life. What's so nice about exercise is that it gives you all these benefits and no downsides, except that it takes time out of your day.

But this is a paradox. Say you spend one hour per day, four

times a week, exercising. You go out for a run, or swim at your local pool. You visit the gym and spend time on the treadmill or step machine, or you pop in your favourite workout video and go at it in your living room. Maybe you bike to work (good for you!) or walk on your lunch hour. Remember that every moment you spend moving your body is beneficial. Studies have shown that there are cumulative benefits to exercising six 10-minute sessions throughout the day (even though the full one-hour session is better).

But getting back to the paradox ... you think to yourself you haven't got four or five hours a week to exercise. And at first, it may cut into your schedule in a measurable way, because you will have to force yourself, and you may feel tired near the beginning of your journey. But after a few weeks, you start to get stronger and your muscles are ever-so-slightly fitter. You "oxygenate" better—that is, your blood carries more oxygen to every part of your body than before, and this becomes more and more the case the longer you exercise and the fitter you become. And, suddenly, you have more energy! Way more than you've ever had! Now, you find you are completing tasks at work and at home in shorter periods of time. You don't have to drag yourself off the couch to get something done, you *spring* off the couch, because your muscles are getting used to being used, and they *like* being used.

Everything takes less time now, and after just a month or so, you're already making up the four hours you exercise in increased efficiency in other areas of your life. Soon, the balance sheet will be on the positive side. You'll be getting so much more done in an average day, in an average week, that the exercise would now be considered a good "risk" by an expert analyst (your return is greater than your investment).

Plus, you are starting to notice something else that doesn't really make itself apparent to your conscious mind until someone points it out or until you cross a personal barrier. *You are thinking more clearly.* Do you know why? For one thing, exercise, as mentioned, enables the blood to carry greater quantities of oxygen. It also increases circulation. Therefore, you are not only getting more oxygen in your blood, but you are also circulating more blood—that is, a greater volume of blood.

Poor circulation is implicated in many common conditions and diseases. These include Alzheimer's disease, liver conditions and diseases, heart and arterial conditions (such as high blood pressure and fatty plaque build-up), headaches (particularly migraines), and the so-called "energy" diseases like fibromyalgia and chronic fatigue syndrome. The reason for this is simple. As you've read elsewhere in this book, the health of your cells—and by extension your entire body—depends on nutrients (from your food) and oxygen being carried to the cells so that they can perform their work. Cells within your blood also have the responsibility of carrying away waste matter. This waste matter filters through your kidneys, liver, and lungs on its way to the "exhaust" systems of the body: your colon, bladder, or respiratory system. The more efficient this system is, the better your body functions.

Claudia Tiefisher:

> Let's use the analogy of the car again. You put clean gas in. You keep the lines that the gas has to travel through free and clear of debris. The gas does its work and, when it has completed this work, the unusable by-products are expelled through the exhaust pipe. If there is a line clogged somewhere or if the engine is performing sluggishly, either not using the fuel correctly or having trouble getting that fuel, then the car performs sluggishly. The same is true if the waste products accumulate in the car. I once had a car whose vacuum seal was working the wrong way. If I made the mistake of starting the car up soon after shutting it off when

the engine was very warm, a spark (which belonged in the tailpipe on its way out of the car) was actually expelling through my engine. One day my battery blew up as a result of this.

In one end and out the other, and efficiency in between.

Have we mentioned the weight loss that will result from exercise? Do you know why excess weight is so detrimental to a person's health? Think again for a moment about the oxygen that your body needs to function. Or, first of all, consider this. Do you remember the last time you walked a long distance carrying something very heavy? Were you out of breath sooner than usual? The reason … okay, this is not rocket science here … is due to the weight you are carrying. So, if you carry a 20-pound sack of flour around with you all the time, it is not unlike carrying 20 extra pounds around your midriff—from an energy expenditure point of view. *However*, having that weight on you as fat is far worse than lugging around a 20-pound sack of flour. This is because your heart has to work that much harder to pump blood through that fat. One pound (half a kilogram) of fat has 8 miles (12 kilometres) of blood vessels. That's a lot of vessels for your heart to pump blood through! Oxygen carries more slowly through fat tissue than it does through muscle tissue, further slowing down the potential efficiency of your circulatory system. The slower this goes, the slower you are to bring needed nutrients and oxygen to all parts of your body, and the slower your body is to remove waste.

Increased circulation is also of benefit to the skin. Skin is another waste disposal site, so the more oxygen you can get near the surface of the skin, the better (oxygen is carried there by the blood). This is why your skin becomes flushed when you exercise hard. The reason your breathing becomes rapid is because the air in your lungs gets used up faster than you can replenish it. The gasping and gulping for air when you have exercised very hard is your body's attempt to refill the lungs with air.

You want this all to take place efficiently, quickly, and cleanly. So how do you make it so? You get fit. And it doesn't take much to get started, but you *must make the start*. And you must stick with it for awhile. Once you're over that 3 or 4-week hump, you likely won't have to drag yourself to the gym or out the door for your run anymore, but until you reach that point, drag yourself. Do whatever it takes. Remember, this is a no-option rule. *You must exercise to achieve optimum health.*

You will find that, if you adopt the principles laid out in this book—in particular making sure your diet is in top form and that you are getting your essential fatty acids—the benefits you derive from exercising will be tripled. You will find it hard to remember the time when you ate corn chips while watching reruns. Now you are out playing with your kids or running a few miles. Your snack food is raw nuts or a banana.

Stick with it. Stick with all of it and you will find new youth in your quest for energy and longevity. Here are some sample programs to get you started moving. First, though, always check with your doctor before starting any exercise program.

For Very Sedentary or Ill Individuals

You say you haven't walked a block in years? You are either very overweight (calculate your body mass index—page 154) or you have suffered from a condition that has kept you bedridden or immobile for a long time. If either of these are the case, you must start with your program very, very slowly.

Week 1 – Start by walking 10 minutes three or four times per day. This could be down to the end of the street you live on and back again. Alternately, get a pass at your local community centre and a few times a week, slip into a bathing suit and take a dip in the pool. For starters, just walk through the pool at the shallow end for 10 or 15 minutes. If you know how to swim, even

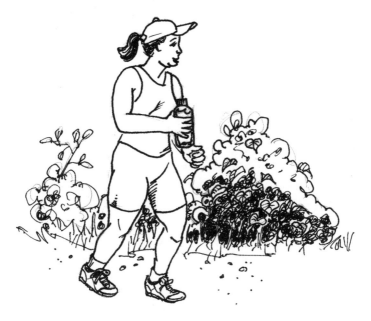

better! Do a few strokes here and there. If you don't know how
to swim, consider taking lessons. Many community centres offer
classes for very overweight people. They are designed to be low
impact (no bouncing or jumping around) and easy on the heart.
Another excellent starter exercise is yoga. One of the benefits of
learning how to move again is learning how to breathe again.
Deep breathing is very important to optimum exercise and also
to vital health.

Week 2 – Stay with your program! You may notice that this week
you really have to drag yourself out the door. It doesn't matter.
Get out that door! If it's raining, grab an umbrella. If it's too hot
outside, make sure you are well hydrated and either change your
exercise time to morning or after sundown. Do not increase the
length of time or the activity level you are engaged in unless you
are really feeling better. It is doubtful that this will be the case
after just one week. In any event, if you do decide to increase

your activity level, do so by no more than 10%—either in distance walked, increased time in the pool, dancing to your favourite music, or time on the stationary bike. Use music to motivate yourself.

Week 3 – Keep it up, you're doing great. This is the last week that you'll feel the urge to flop on the couch instead of getting out and moving your body. No matter what age you are, and no matter what your fitness goals, you should also be thinking about doing at least a little bit of weight training. This is especially important for women, as women lose one pound of muscle each year starting at age 35. So, go to any fitness store or to a larger variety store, and buy yourself a small set of weights. The smallest should be about a pound, and there are nice ones you can get; they're not like little dumbbells, they're little bags of sand with a Velcro strap attached that you can wrap around your hand. Carrying these while you walk will increase the benefits of any walking exercise you do, as it will burn more calories and increase aerobic (oxygen) output.

Week 4 – You can slowly increase your workout time and/or distance now. Still, you don't want to overdo it at any point. The top two reasons people quit their workout routine is injury and expecting too much, too soon. It takes a long time to get fit. It took a long time to put on those extra pounds and, unfortunately, it will take even longer to take them off. We've talked at length about how weight gain and loss work in the chapters on weight loss and understanding fats. However, there is still one simple rule that can't be denied or argued. One pound of fat is equal to 3,500 calories. This means you have to consume 3,500 fewer calories than you expend, or work off 3,500 calories, in order to lose one pound.

Safe weight loss is approximately one pound a week or even less. Remember, the faster you take the weight off, the less likely you are to keep it off. Remember, too, that you are exercising (and eating right) *for life*. This is not something you are doing in preparation for an upcoming high school reunion or family wedding so you can fit into that special dress. As a matter of fact, rapid, frequent weight gain and loss are very, very hard on the body. Take the weight off slowly, gradually, and keep it off by always eating sensibly. You will add immeasurable energy and pleasure to your life and years of active living when you reach your senior years.

Week 5 – It's not a bad idea to seek the advice of a fitness expert at this point. You may certainly be increasing the time and/or distance you exercise by 10% every week, if you feel comfortable doing that. Start to sign up for longer or slightly harder classes, but don't jump into an advanced step class if you are severely overweight or have had knee surgery. Remember, once again, the lessons this book is attempting to teach: *balance and common sense*. A healthy dose of both will bring you health and keep you healthy.

If you were walking 10 minutes four times daily the first week and 15 minutes 3 times a day the second week and so on, you may be ready now to walk a full 30 minutes. If you get tired and can't do this, though, stop. And if it hurts, you should also stop. One of the most damaging sayings ever to make it into mainstream popular culture years back was, "No pain, no gain." This is absolutely not true. When you get very, very fit—to the point where you will want to run marathons and so on—there will certainly be times when you will experience what is known as "muscle burn". You will come to love this feeling when you get there because accompanying it, invariably, is a feeling of having achieved a personal best and *knowing* you are stretching yourself.

   Olympic athletes were not made on haphazard schedules.
                                                    — source unknown

Possibly the most important thing in helping you to achieve and maintain your fitness goals is to have your goals written down and to have them be as specific as possible. And not only your goals, but the steps you must take to achieve those goals. This is true whether it is to complete a marathon that is taking place in six months, or simply to lose a few pounds. It is also true if your doctor has told you that you are at high risk for diabetes or heart disease, and that you must trim 50 pounds and watch your intake of saturated fat. Perhaps you simply want to be lean and trim so that when you are shopping for clothes you can buy an item that really strikes your fancy, instead of one that "doesn't make my tummy look like it sticks out very much."

For instance, let's say you are in good health, but you are 30 pounds overweight. You decide to begin a walk/run program. But have you decided when you will begin? Tomorrow? Next week? On the 15th of next month? Have you decided how many times a week you will do this? Will you vaguely decide three or four is good, then only achieve it once or twice? Have you decided which days you will do it, and at what times? Have you decided where you will run, how long you will run, and how much of the distance will be spent walking, and how much of it running? Write each of these specifics down.

Your goal might look like this: I want to lose 30 pounds. Starting next Sunday, I will run/walk every Sunday, Monday, Wednesday, Friday, and Saturday. I will run at 7:00 in the morning and I will follow this specified route. I have a sportswatch on which I will time myself. The run is 30 minutes in length. I will warm up with 2 minutes of brisk walking, followed by 30 seconds of running, and 90 seconds of walking. I will continue this until I come home. I will record my time to monitor my progress. I will increase each week's sessions by no more than 10% either in distance or time.

Now you have a goal. It is specific and written down. No excuses or vagueness can creep in. You know what you are doing.

Sedentary Individuals in Good Health

If you are in good health but simply haven't moved your body in quite a while and feel you are out of shape, you may start at a higher level than the previous one discussed. Again, it is vital to see your doctor before embarking on any exercise program, and also to take into consideration personal truths. Are you a morning person or evening person? Schedule your exercise accordingly. Can you motivate yourself to exercise on your own, or should you join a gym and be around others? Do you hate running? Then don't do it. Choose swimming, walking, or skiing instead. Do you have problems with your feet that are aggravated by the pounding of running or step classes? Then stick to lower-impact exercises. For cardiovascular health, use a step or rowing machine or stationary bicycle. Take all of these factors into consideration when you (and/or your personal trainer) design a fitness program geared specifically for your needs.

Design a program that stretches your abilities slightly but that doesn't push you too much. The key is to listen to your body. A good beginning running program, for example, might be the specific goal outlined above. When you can do this comfortably, without huffing and puffing too much, increase the distance you cover. You should increase distance as opposed to trying to cover the same distance in less time. You should be exercising for at least 30 minutes each time you go out.

If you prefer not to time yourself as you run, pick distance markers or just listen to your body. This last can be tough to do, however, because it's harder to measure progress and more difficult to push yourself. You're more likely to stop when you could do more; you're more likely to push yourself when you should be slowing down.

An excellent way to get into exercising long-term, especially if you have no routine at the moment, is to set your sights on a sanctioned 5K or 10K walk or run. If you pick a run that is, say, five months in the future, work backwards from the date. This way, you can know exactly where you need to be each week. Again, don't push yourself. The quickest way to giving up is by overdoing it. And, if you injure yourself, you'll also be sidelined.

Warm-Up and Cool-Down

No matter what sport you choose to play, or what activity you decide to participate in, warm up your muscles with gentle stretching and gentle movement before you begin. Talk to a qualified sports person like a therapist or trainer to determine what sort of warm-up you should be doing for your particular activity. You should spend about 10 minutes warming up.

At the end of your workout routine, when your muscles are warm, is the best time to engage in real stretching. Be careful when you stretch, however. Never bounce—this is the "old" way and has been found to be damaging. Instead, reach slowly through your stretch until you feel discomfort in the stretched muscle, and hold for 10 to 30 seconds. Repeat. Be careful how you stretch your back—it is easy to pull a muscle here and this will sideline you for days, perhaps weeks.

Exercise Myths

1. *Sit-ups are best done with someone holding your feet down.* Not true. In fact, sit-ups shouldn't even be done to the full sitting up position. You only need to achieve, at most, a 45 degree angle. Lift and lower slowly, never jerk; knees are slightly bent. Alternately, you can place your feet flat against a wall at the same level as your knees. This makes the exercise harder, but more effective. To stretch out sore tummy muscles from doing sit-ups, rotate your bent legs from the hip (you are still lying down) sideways onto the mat, keeping your knees together. Stretch to both sides.

2. *You should "spot reduce" if you have trouble spots on your body.* Spot reducing isn't even possible. When you work specific muscles or muscle groups with specific exercises or weight lifting,

you will sculpt those muscles. They change shape—becoming longer or larger. If you have a tummy from overeating, or big hips or a large *derriere*, you will not make them smaller by lifting weights aimed at the muscles that are in that area of your body. You will tone the muscles, but the fat on top will stay there, unless you burn calories—do aerobic exercise—to reduce overall body fat.

3. *When you exercise, you turn fat into muscle.* No you don't. Muscle is muscle and fat is fat. You can develop, strengthen, tone, and elongate muscles, sculpting your body into pleasing and healthy shapes, but fat will always stay fat. You either have that fat or you don't have it. If you have too much body fat, you must burn it off. Then the muscles underneath have a chance to show through.

4. *You should work out every day.* You don't need to work out every day, nor should you. Weight training, in particular, requires you to take regular breaks. For instance, you might have a program where you work your upper body muscles twice a week and your lower body muscles twice a week. You should alternate which group of muscles you work on. When you lift weights, you are actually microscopically tearing muscle fiber. When the muscle repairs itself—*the next day, when the muscle is at rest*—it becomes every-so-slightly larger for the next "assault"—i.e., the next time you tax that muscle by lifting heavy weights with it. The same is true for cardiovascular exercise. You should rest a couple of days every week, or at the very least one.

5. *The heavier the weight, the better it is.* Lifting heavy weights for fewer reps builds strength; lifting lighter weights more often (i.e., more sets and/or more repetitions) builds endurance. Which program you do depends on your fitness goals. Talk to a qualified expert.

6. *You can lift any old thing to build muscles.* Do not use milk jugs or phone books as weights you "lift". You stand a good chance of hurting yourself because the balance of the weight is all wrong. Your wrists, for example, would be the most prone to injury.

7. *You can't be fit unless you exercise.* Though this "myth" appears to fly in the face of everything discussed so far in this chapter, it's true that a person can be incredibly fit without doing "exercise" as we know it, of any kind. These are people with very physical jobs, where all day long they are on their feet, lifting, hoisting, carrying, walking, standing. Or they are people who have been into sports from a young age and well into their adulthood continue to be involved in sports of every kind. People like this wouldn't be required to start a jogging regimen or a workout schedule at the gym. Having said this, though, it wouldn't hurt them if they did. They'd simply be fitter still.

8. *I'm not seeing any results, so I should change what I'm doing, or drastically increase what I'm doing.* Not necessarily so. First of all, never drastically increase the difficulty or duration of your workout. Change should always be gradual. Secondly, if you are uttering this in the first couple of months of getting active, you are expecting too much, too soon. Remember, you should do enough that you are stretching yourself slightly with each workout. But the emphasis is on the word *slightly*. Stretch yourself, yes. There's no point in going out for a run that does not elevate your heart rate at all—you get very little aerobic benefit from such a workout. However, don't push yourself until you are in pain or unable to move the next day.

9. *I can get fit by working out only on the weekends.* You are more likely to injure yourself than get fit by engaging in sudden bursts of activities on your two days off. You should exercise a minimum of four days per week, preferably five.

10. *I'm thin, so I don't need to work out.* Just because you aren't overweight does not mean you are fit. Check muscle tone and endurance—do you have enough of both? Could you run a mile? Swim several laps? Can you keep up with your kids, your spouse? Could you dance all night? Do you sleep well at night? How's your level of energy all day long? Do you have a good appetite? These are questions you need to ask yourself if you think you can get away without engaging in physical activity.

Claudia Tiefisher:

> I started my running on a routine similar to the one described above. In the course of writing this book, I do not think I could have managed the stress that went along with the deadlines had I not been running. There are days I don't feel like going, but I remind myself how incredible I'll feel when I get back home. One of the more interesting things I've noticed in my fitness journey, is that there really is a sizable psychological factor that affects your exercising.

> I start off with brisk walking before I start to jog. My first couple of jogging intervals are at a slower pace than subsequent ones. My run takes me around the valley in which we live (out in the country). On the way back (the road goes around in a loop), it is slightly uphill, and I always predict that it will be difficult, seeing how it is near the end of my run. Strangely enough, it never is. Either I have more energy at this point in my run than I am giving myself credit for (meaning I need to push myself just a little bit harder), or the fact that I am near the end of the run is giving me a psychological push. Either way, how well I perform, and how difficult I think it will be, seems to be totally in my mind.

I have to say that I have never felt better. Exercise is so very, very important. Please, do whatever it takes to move your body. Regularly.

Dr. Bill Code:

I have started running many times in my life and have lasted up to six weeks. Usually I only make it two or three weeks. Walking or cycling to and from work have been my best success. The most important thing is a lasting lifestyle change. Erratic, rare exercise efforts risk injury and provide very little benefit. Do something with people you care about and you will enhance each other's enthusiasm. Evening or morning walks (Bob Hope described golf as a great excuse for a walk) are inexpensive, easy, and good for your relationships. Your exercise will get you fitter, reduce your stress levels, and help you lose weight. Emu oil will enhance your comfort from aches and pains and increase your chances of continuing. Professional athletes use emu oil and other assorted devices—why not you?

Emu Oil & Exercise

Emu oil has critical, valuable essential fatty acids (EFAs) in it for optimal recovery of the body from exercise. You'll read in the next section how emu oil's makeup is very close to that of human skin. You'll also read about its anti-inflammatory properties. What this means is that if you have sore muscles at the end of the day or the end of a workout, you can rub some emu oil on the sore area and you will experience deep relief. Emu oil decreases stiffness and soreness and sometimes prevents them from happening altogether. It's possible the way it does this is to speed up recovery from lactic acid build-up. It is great for blisters on the feet (apply some emu oil, put a band-aid on and leave overnight).

Internally, emu oil capsules will provide the essential fatty acids necessary for proper energy transfer between cells in your body, thereby facilitating higher metabolism. Okay, we need to back up and describe what happens when you respire (breathe)—taking in oxygen and expelling carbon dioxide—the most basic component of life itself.

Oxygen accounts for 20% of the air around us. Oxygen molecules breathed in are in the O_2 format (two molecules of oxygen bound to each other). They travel in through the mouth or nose, into the windpipe (or trachea), and down into the lungs. There it is exchanged at the membrane of the *alveoli*, which is the interface between the gas side and the bloodstream side of the lungs. It crosses the membrane into the bloodstream, where it is partly dissolved in the blood. Mostly, though, oxygen is carried around the body by hemoglobin. Hemoglobin picks up oxygen at a high oxygen tension and then drops it off at a lower oxygen tension. What this means is that where oxygen is high, such as in the lungs, it goes onto hemoglobin, riding on it, just like a little cart. It is then dropped off at the capillaries at the tissue end—for example at the tips of your fingers, the tips of your feet, or in your critical organs, where oxygen tensions are low.

Oxygen primarily goes to the specialty organs such as the heart, lungs, brain, kidney, and liver. The rest goes to muscles when they're exercising and working hard. The oxygen is dropped off there, goes into the body's biochemical pathway, and is then used in the cells to burn up the food that we've taken in (this is called *metabolism*). The food we've taken in was based on carbon—whether it was carbohydrate, protein, fats, or alcohol. The body takes that and uses it (burns it). In the process, the oxygen becomes bound to one of the carbons that are used from the burnt up group, and then becomes carbon dioxide.

Carbon dioxide, interestingly enough, is partly dissolved in the blood. Mostly, though, it now attaches to hemoglobin, travels back to the lungs, crosses the membrane of the alveoli, up into the windpipe, and out through the mouth and nose (this function is all driven by the pumping of the heart).

Whenever we use our muscles, we have increased oxygen demand. That's where the term *aerobic exercise* comes from. *Aerobic* exercise takes place as long as we're able to get oxygen into the lungs quickly enough to maintain continuous aerobic oxygenation (or supply of oxygen to the muscles and tissues). When we go beyond the body's ability to keep up (when we can't breathe fast enough), we then go into *anaerobic* (without oxygen) oxygenation or supply. This is where there is not enough oxygen to go through each of the molecules of fat or protein or carbohydrate that are being burned up. When this happens, we form something called *lactic acid*. Lactic acid is the breakdown product that is produced when there isn't enough oxygen to look after the pathways. So, when you run a 100 yard dash, you may well start out with aerobic oxygenation, but you will primarily end up being in lactic acid production from anaerobic oxygenation.

This brings up the importance of exercising in a range where oxygenation is always present. While lactic acid isn't dangerous in the short term, it will cause cramping, pain, and stiffness in the muscles. Anaerobic exercise also means you are not burning very many calories (anaerobic means burning without oxygen). We cannot sustain anaerobic exercise for very long.

A Cross-Canada Story

Meet Pierre Doré. Pierre bicycled all across Canada—a distance of 8,000 km —from Mile 0 in Victoria, B.C., starting June 1, 1998, finishing August 31, 1998. The trip got him into the Guinness Book of World Records.

Dr. Bill Code:
> Pierre was 34 years old the spring of 1998. We met on the Vicky Gabereau show. I was there talking about emu oil and he was there talking about his primarily

wooden, recumbent bicycle. He also spoke of his energy and enthusiasm to promote the Trans-Canada Trail. He'd arranged to stay in International Hostels as he cycled across Canada. His story intrigued me and he was in need of sponsorship so we decided to team up.

We set him up with a number of emu farmers and emu oil promoters across the country. He did so many TV and radio spots promoting the trip that he was hoarse with laryngitis prior to an interview in Saskatchewan. It was Pierre himself who thought of gargling with emu oil. It worked miraculously well; he was able to speak without problems during the interview. Since then, several of us, including myself a number of times, have had problems with laryngitis. An emu oil gargle seems to solve this problem.

Pierre used emu oil instead of sunscreen on his body for the three-month duration of the trip. He never had a sunburn; instead, he got a beautiful tan.[1] He also used it exclusively on his bicycle chain as a lubricant. Following the trip I bought the bicycle that has that chain on it—the one he started with and went all across Canada with. In addition to all its other uses, emu oil appears to be an amazing industrial lubricant as well.

Pierre was out of shape and somewhat pot-bellied before he started on this cross-Canada trip. He'd done almost no training, and the route, of course, starts in the mountains as soon as you leave Vancouver. His solution for aches and pains or stiffness at night or in the morning was to rub emu oil on his muscles and joints.

When he finished his journey in St. John's, Newfoundland, Pierre was more fit and stronger—and healthier—than ever. At this time, Pierre is planning an even greater, more challenging journey on a newly designed recumbent bike.

In Summary

Exercise will benefit every area of your life. If you get your body moving and adopt the other principles we've put forward in this book, your quality of life will improve immeasurably. You need not become a marathon runner, nor a long-distance cyclist like Pierre. Just stick with it. Make it a part of your lifestyle. You'll be happy you did.

Body Mass Index

The Body Mass Index is a scientific way to determine how overweight you are (it also shows underweight). Here's how you work it out:

Take your weight in kilograms and divide by your height squared in metres. For example, if you weigh 75 kg and are 1.69 metres (169 centimetres) tall, the equation looks like this:

$$\frac{75 \text{ kilograms}}{1.69 \times 1.69 \text{ meters}}$$

= 75 divided by 2.856 = 26.26
(use an electronic calculator)

To figure out in pounds and inches, one kg equals .45 pounds and one centimetre equals 2.54 centimetres

In the example above, the body mass index is 26. For males, this is just entering the overweight range. For females, it is considered overweight. A female's BMI should fall between 19 and 25 depending on build. A male's BMI should fall between 20 and 26. Overweight is considered between the upper limit of BMI and 29. Over 29 is considered obese.

CHAPTER 6

Supplementation for Optimal Nutrition and Prevention of Disease

Nutrition supplementation has become a burgeoning industry. Why has this occurred? We believe it is a shift in people's mindsets. Many of us, especially the well-informed, are now aiming for wellness and optimal health. It is now felt that 70 per cent of our chronic health problems are nutrition based. In this chapter, we outline three food pyramids to permit readers to see how we should be changing the emphasis from disease to wellness. The RDA (Recommended Dietary Allowance) background is next. Following this is a "capsule" summary of the vitamins and minerals and other supplements our bodies can benefit from.

First, the three different food pyramids. The "Official" USDA Food Pyramid suggests we emphasize breads, cereals, rice, and pasta the most. This is based more on what we need to eat to prevent illness. North Americans have continued to gain weight and develop more chronic illness than ever before. The "Mediterranean" Food Pyramid is from a cultural group that has less heart disease than we have in North America. The greatest change here is the emphasis on olive oil, a monounsaturated fatty acid.

The third and perhaps ultimate is the "Optimal Nutrition" Food Pyramid. It is designed by Roy Walford in his book

Beyond the 120 Year Diet[1]. All three pyramids are shown on the page opposite *(figure 6-1).*

Walford has shifted fruits, vegetables, beans, and nuts to the anchor or dominant position. Carbohydrates are assigned a position on a *glycemic index* (or GI). Glycemic index is a combination of carbohydrates' absorption and how high an insulin release they cause. Foods that are low in *complex* carbohydrates and high in *simple* carbohydrates, like donuts, would be assigned a high GI. Foods like broccoli, apples, whole wheat bread, and brown rice would be assigned a low GI.

The vast majority of carbohydrates consumed should be in the low to medium GI range. Refined foods and simple carbohydrates trigger a high GI. Avoid simple sugars and refined foods. Reach for whole grains and whole grain products whenever you can. Walford also puts selected supplements at the top. He recognizes many or most of us are unable to obtain all of our body's needs from food readily available to us. We agree with him. We should all eat according to his food pyramid and take vitamin, mineral, and other supplements regularly.

Finally, it takes five to six times as much nutrition to *reverse* a condition that's already in place, as it does to *prevent* problems.

Genetically, humans are "old" beings—we probably haven't changed for hundreds of thousands of years. Our diet, by comparison, has changed drastically in just the last 10,000 years with the agricultural revolution, the discovery of fire, and the fact that we are now living on the majority of the earth's surface. All these changes have an impact on our dietary requirements and on what our dietary intakes should be. It is thought that 10,000 years ago, over the course of a year, we ate some 200 different seeds, nuts, fruits, and other foods. Today, we would be hard pressed to name more than 20 major foods in our diets. Most of these are based on wheat, rice, soy, corn, milk products, and a number of common vegetables—especially in North America— such as peas, beans, carrots, and corn. Further limiting variety is

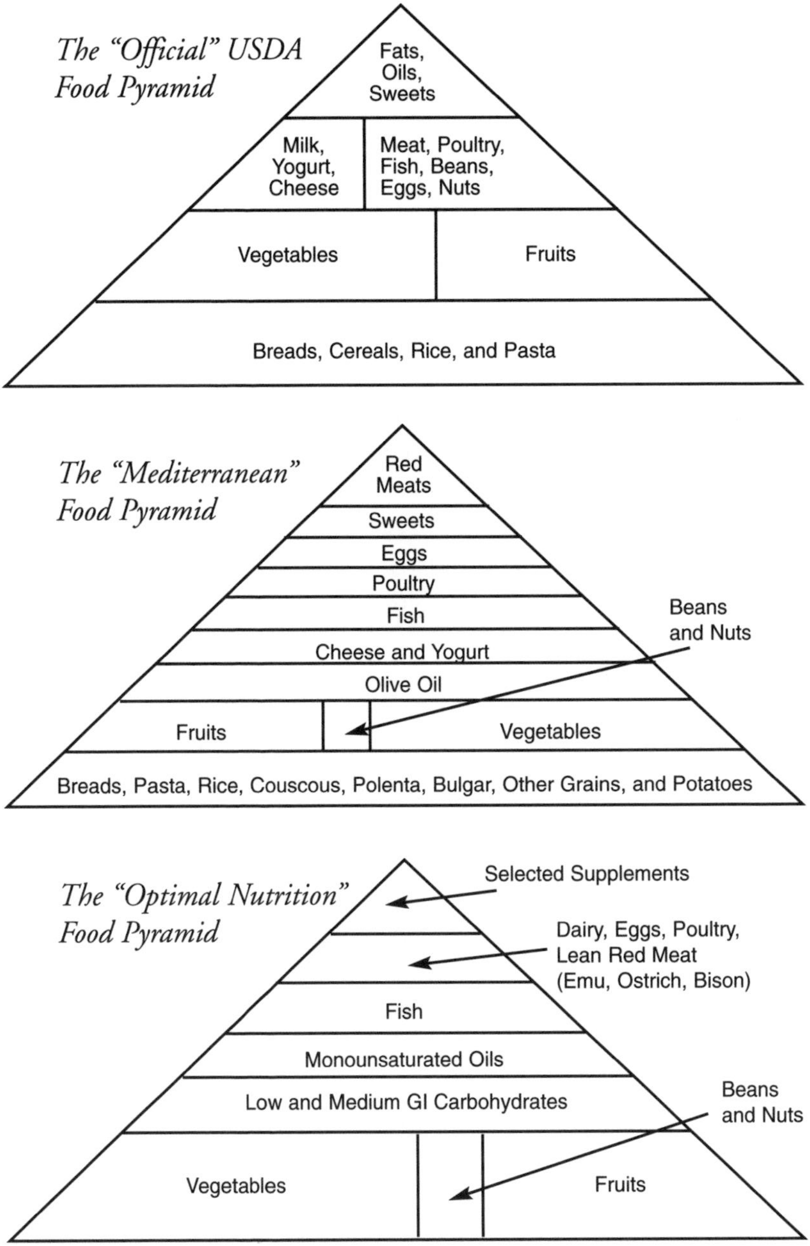

Figure 6-1: The Three Pyramids as described by Walford[1]

the fact that we can get most foods all year long by importing them from elsewhere. This often results in our eating a single variety of fruit or vegetable (for instance, only iceberg lettuce or Granny Smith apples).

All of these factors have made a difference. One of the other features of our modern life is that we have moved to more temperate climates, that is, further away from the equator. This has impacted on us as well, because most of us now live in areas where we can't make much vitamin D from the sun.

Recommended Daily Allowances (RDAs)

RDAs were set by the Committee on Dietary Allowances of the National Academy of Sciences. Over time, these have become almost sacrosanct. The knowledge base for these nutritional estimates was based on six criteria:

1. The amount of the particular nutrient that healthy people consume.
2. The amount needed to avoid a particular disease (e.g., scurvy was very common and the recommended daily allowance of vitamin C is enough to prevent scurvy).
3. The degree of tissue saturation or the adequacy of body function in relation to that nutrient intake.
4. Nutrient balance studies that measure nutritional status in relation to intake.
5. Studies of volunteers experimentally maintained on diets deficient in a nutrient, followed by their improvement, or signs of deficiency going away, when a certain amount of the nutrient is resupplied.
6. Extrapolation from animal experiments in which deficiencies have been produced by exclusion of a single nutrient from the diet.

A seventh criteria can be considered, and this is what we would like to focus on as well. This criteria looks at longevity and disease information.[2]

Listed in this chapter are the "official" RDA or DRI (daily recommended intake) levels of several important vitamins, minerals and other nutritional supplements. Listed below the RDA/DRI is the supplementation level the authors suggest. These amounts are *total* daily amounts. In many cases, we also list a "treatment" level, which will apply to some individuals.

Fat-Soluble Vitamins

Vitamin A
    RDA/DRI   5,000 IU (for men) 4,000 IU (for women)
    Supplement[3] 5,000 IU (for men) 4,000 IU (for women)
                         (4,000 IU pregnancy / planning pregnancy)

Treatment notes: beta carotene is safest—the body can convert it to vitamin A
Toxicity Level: more than 50,000 IU per day, over several years
Comparison: 10,000 IU equals 25 mg
Special Considerations: Vitamin A excess in pregnancy can contribute to birth defects. Only 4,000 IU per day should be consumed. Women should stay off the acne drug Accutane if pregnant or planning on becoming pregnant.
Best Sources of beta carotene: carrots, apricots, mangoes, yams, squash, grapefruit, broccoli, spinach, green peppers, cantaloupe, watermelon, tomatoes and tomato products, pumpkin, orange juice
Best Sources of vitamin A: liver, kidney, butter, whole milk, fortified low fat and skim milk

We should be able to obtain the recommended amount of vitamin A from food sources. It is almost impossible to exceed the safe level of vitamin A if we use the forerunner *beta carotene*, from which the body can make vitamin A. The safest way to supplement vitamin A is to make sure you get plenty of beta carotene. Beta carotene is non-toxic and the body will only make as much vitamin A from it as it needs. For general health, a daily supplement of 25,000 IU beta carotene is reasonable.

Vitamin D

RDA/DRI   same for men and women
200 IU (under age 50)
400 IU (over age 50)
600 IU (over age 70)

Supplement   1,000 IU all age groups, both men and women, including the amount from milk and sunlight

Treatment notes: dosage is 4,000 IU
Toxicity Level: 10,000 IU
Best Sources: cod liver oil, herring oil, cooked Pacific oysters, salmon oil, canned mackerel, fortified fluid milks (including cow's milk, soy and rice milks)

Vitamin D is harder to get from food than vitamin A. Despite the upper limit safety range stated above, it is probably very safe up to 40,000 units. There is only one recorded case of signs of toxicity at 10,000 units.[4]

If we lived at the equator and ran around naked, we would make about 10,000 units per day. At the 49th parallel, however, we only get sunshine at the correct angle four to six months of the year. A certain angle of light on exposed skin is required for the ultraviolet rays to convert the precursor (from cholesterol) into the early forms of vitamin D.

We believe 4,000 units per day is an optimum amount for therapy of autoimmune problems such as multiple sclerosis. Vitamin D is so important because of its autoimmune stabilizing capabilities and, because it's a hormone, it works on the immune system as a modulator.

This is one example where we may need to take more to reverse a condition that has taken hold, than we do to actually have optimal health. Other autoimmune illnesses where vitamin D intake should be increased: osteoarthritis, rheumatoid arthritis, and inflammatory bowel diseases (including Crohn's disease and ulcerative colitis). Psoriasis and asthma may also benefit from vitamin D supplementation.

The RDA for vitamin D is enough to prevent deficiency diseases such as rickets. Of course, vitamin D has importance far beyond rickets. One of these, as we've talked about, is its role in the immune system as a modulator. Of considerable interest, too, is that vitamin D is thought to help prevent cancers. No one really knows why, though there are three theories as to how this might work.

One of the theories is that vitamin D kills cells which contain DNA mutations. Another theory talks about vitamin D somehow recognizing and promoting the death of unusual, mutated, or cancer-type cells. The final theory is that vitamin D actually promotes protein transcription (meaning that we can make proteins from a gene that is one of the body's cancer watchdogs).

Vitamin D has been added to milk since the 1950's in order to prevent rickets. Interestingly, milk protein (albumin) is similar in structure to vitamin D receptors in the body. This represents a potential problem. An immune reaction against the milk protein could also result in a reaction against the vitamin D receptor. This would reduce the ability of vitamin D to bind to the receptors on the cells. Vitamin D is then unable to do its important functions in bone cells or in the immune system. Another important point is that many people are unaware that other milk products such as ice cream, yogurt, and cheese do not have vitamin D added to them.

Only about 10 to 20 minutes per day out of doors without sunscreen should be adequate for vitamin D development. However, the unfortunate reality is that we lose this ability as we get older. By the time we are 70 years of age, our ability to make vitamin D from sunlight is 70% reduced. Also, the further north we live, the less likely it is we are going to get adequate ultraviolet rays from the sun.

People who primarily work indoors may not get the sunshine even in those magical four months. People with MS usually avoid the heat, and as such are even less likely to get it. With the increasing use of sunscreens, we are getting less and less vitamin D all the time. For example, an SPF 8 sunscreen reduces your vitamin D production by 95%. An SPF 30 cuts it to zero. It is indeed a conundrum. What should we do? The safe thing is to take a supplement. Going to the tanning salons for sunshine and vitamin D is no substitute for real sunshine. You shouldn't be under a tanning lamp for more than 5 to 10 minutes per day anyway. Any more will result in injury to the skin.

The recommended form to supplement with is vitamin D3, which is another name for *1,25-dihydroxycholecalciferol* or *calcitriol*. This form of vitamin D is the most active.

Vitamin E

RDA/DRI	22 IU from natural sources (for both men and women)
Supplement	400 IU for both men and women

Treatment notes: 800-1,600 IU will help most individuals slow or reverse atherosclerosis and heart disease
Toxicity Level: 2,000 IU
Special Considerations: We suggest a combination of d-alpha, d-gamma, and tocotrienol (check the label of your vitamin E product).
Best Sources: Mostly found in vegetable and seed oils, nuts and seeds, and green and leafy green vegetables. Especially good sources are wheat germ oil, sunflower and safflower oil, peanuts, almonds and soybean, corn and canola oils

Vitamin E is an important antioxidant. Supplementation is

now routinely recommended to patients with Alzheimer's disease. While the vitamin will not reverse or halt the disease, it will slow its progression.

Is there a difference between natural and synthetic vitamin E? Yes. Natural vitamins are absorbed into the bloodstream twice as fast as the synthetic form.[5] The natural form of vitamin E can be recognized by the letter d-, as in d-alpha-tocopherol.

Vitamin K

RDA/DRI   80 micrograms (for men)
                     65 micrograms (for women)
                     in individuals aged 25 years and over
Supplement   400 micrograms total, including all food
                     sources and supplemental

Treatment notes: 800-1,000 micrograms/day to reduce osteoporosis and also excessive menstrual bleeding
Toxicity Level: very high at 30 mg, or no toxicity
Comparison: 1,000 micrograms = 1 mg
Special Considerations: see below re: Warfarin (Coumadin)
Best Sources: high in spinach, Brussels sprouts, broccoli, and green leaf lettuce

The "K" comes the Danish word for coagulation, spelled *koagulation*. Vitamin K is needed by the liver to make six of our blood clotting proteins. It is also essential for the synthesis of osteocalcin, the protein in bone tissue.

Warfarin (Coumadin) stops the liver synthesis of blood clotting proteins. Hence, changes in the diet of vitamin K foods can alter this Warfarin-induced blood thinning. If you are on this drug, try to keep your diet relatively consistent. That way you can have varying amounts of vitamin K and other substances that may interfere with the drug, but you stay within a consistent range. This makes it easier for you and your physician to determine what dosage you should be taking.

Water-Soluble Vitamins

Vitamin C
    RDA/DRI   90 mg (for men)   75 mg (for women)
                     Smokers add 35 mg/day
    Supplement   500-1,000 mg (both men and women)

Toxicity Level: 2-4 grams (long-term use)
Best Sources: Good sources of vitamin C include vegetables, especially broccoli, peppers, potatoes (not just the skin!), Brussels sprouts, sour cherries, cranberries, plums, and of course citrus fruits. Vitamin C in any of these breaks down on air contact, so the fresher, the better.

Humans are one of the few animals unable to make vitamin C from sunshine on our skin. Vitamin C is also our most popular vitamin supplement and yet also the most controversial. Everyone agrees, however, that vitamin C is essential. A deficiency results in the "sailor's illness"—scurvy. Scurvy results in bleeding gums, poor wound healing and bruising easily.

If you have determined you need more than an average amount of antioxidants, vitamin C is the best water-soluble circulating antioxidant known. If there is an excess of it, it is literally dumped out by the kidneys.

Vitamin C has a fairly short "active" time in the body. Therefore, you may want to take it on a four-times-a-day basis. Vitamin C supplementation is important if you're going to have surgery or other interventions, or if you must take a course of drugs. If you are cleansing your liver or other organs, losing body fat, or if you have mercury fillings, vitamin C will work to counter the effects of these.

In his book *Real Age*[6], Dr. Roizen suggests you might consider eating some fruit or taking vitamin C one to two hours before exercise. This is because exercise can cause buildup of some free radicals, and of course vitamin C is one of our favourite antioxidants. Also, if you're an individual who experiences stomach upset from straight ascorbic acid (vitamin C), then you might consider taking calcium ascorbate. This is another form of vitamin C, and is also a source of calcium. Vitamin C provides a healthy base for the walls of blood vessels, repairing them when they become damaged. Other benefits of vitamin C are helping to lower blood pressure, helping to prevent cataracts, enhancing healing, and is very important in the forming of collagen.

Vitamin B Group

Thiamin (Vitamin B1)
RDA/DRI   1.2 mg (for men)   1.1 mg (for women)
                      1.5 mg (pregnant or breastfeeding)
Supplement   RDA levels are adequate

Treatment notes: see text, especially important in alcoholic withdrawal and ongoing alcoholism
Toxicity Level: 50 mg, but may be much higher, as kidney can readily dispose of any extra of this water-soluble vitamin
Best Sources: soy beans, brown rice, sunflower seeds, peanuts, brewer's yeast, wheat germ, pork, fish, enriched grain products, cooked dried beans and peas

Because of the high incidence of this vitamin in most whole grains, supplementation isn't required. However, you will likely find B1 together with the other B vitamins in most B-complex vitamin formulas.

If the supplement amount is based on B-complex vitamin mixtures, then our guideline is 50-100 mg per day. Treatment to prevent deficiency is especially important in diabetes, multiple sclerosis, Crohn's disease, and other brain illnesses (e.g., epilepsy patients on Dilantin). Mental function in Alzheimer's disease and senility shows improvement with 3 to 8 grams per day.[7]

Riboflavin (Vitamin B2)
RDA/DRI   1.3 mg (for men)   1.1 mg (for women)
Supplement   5-10 mg per day

Treatment notes: To prevent migraine headaches, 400 mgs per day suggested
Toxicity Level: 500 mg daily long-term, but no toxicity reported
Special Considerations: Excess riboflavin may speed cataract growth
Best Sources: liver, almonds, mushrooms, whole grains, leafy green vegetables, and soybeans.

Niacin (Vitamin B3)
RDA/DRI   16 mg (for men)   14 mg (for women)
Supplement   100-300 mg per day

Comparison: 1,000 mg = 1 gram (g)
Treatment notes: 100 mg three times a day and increase over 4-6 weeks to therapeutic dose of 1.5 g/day
Toxicity Level: 3-4 grams per day, with no serious effects[8]
Considerations: People who are pregnant, suffer from diabetes, glaucoma, gout, liver disease, or peptic ulcers should use niacin supplements with caution.
Best Sources: liver, eggs, fish, peanuts, legumes, whole grains, avocadoes, milk. Other sources are broccoli, brewer's yeast, cheese, corn flour, pork, potatoes, tomatoes, wheat germ, and whole wheat products

Niacin is used to treat *hypercholesterolemia* or other *hyperlipidemias.* Dosages to treat these conditions are 1 to 3 grams per day. This dosage can be toxic to the liver, however, so supplementation at this range should be done only under the advice of a physician. In addition, high levels of niacin cause severe flushing in some individuals and must be discontinued or taken at a much lower dose. High fiber is probably a safer, healthier way to reduce cholesterol and low density lipoproteins.

Folic Acid (Vitamin B4) (also called folate)

RDA/DRI   400 micrograms (0.4 mg) (men and women)
              600 micrograms (0.6 mg)
              (pregnancy/planning pregnancy)
Supplement 400 micrograms (0.4) per day

Treatment notes: Increase to 10 mg/day to treat cervical dysplasia (abnormal pap smear) and depression. Do not take high doses of this vitamin unless you are sure you are not deficient in vitamin B12.
Toxicity Level: 200 mg daily
Best Sources: Green leafy vegetables, broccoli, cabbage, legumes, asparagus, oranges, root vegetables, and whole grains.

There is good evidence that many of us may be deficient in this vitamin. It's best to supply it regularly in the diet, particularly for women who are considering getting pregnant. Folic acid reduces the incidence of neural tube defects, also known as spina bifida, in infants. Folic acid also plays an important role with regard to placement of calcium in the body. It is very important in cell division because it is needed in DNA synthesis.

Another issue that's very important is that folate will reduce one of the recognized risk factors of heart disease—the build-up of homocysteine.[9] When you consume the amino acid methionine, it is converted into homocysteine for transport to the liver. Homocysteine is somewhat toxic, but in the liver it's converted into methionine or cysteine, which are both used in liver detoxification.[10] However, a build-up of homocysteine can occur, which leads to hardening of the arteries and heart disease. This is particularly the case if your liver enzymes are not working in top form. Supplementation with folic acid, vitamin B6, and vitamin B12 can bring homocysteine levels back down.

Routinely, as we age, folic acid concentrations drop. It is the most common vitamin deficiency found in older people (over half the U.S. population does not get enough per day). The average intake is approximately 275 micrograms per day from diet. Therefore, a 400 micrograms per day supplement would be reasonable. This alone could reduce heart attacks in North America by 10 per cent.

If you take a folic acid supplement, you should also take vitamin B12. Folic acid supplementation can mask a vitamin B12 deficiency. Vitamin B12 deficiency can result in nerve damage, which cannot be reversed.

Pantothenic Acid (Vitamin B5)
RDA/DRI None established
Supplement 500 mg per day (both men and women)

Toxicity Level: very high at 3,000 mg
Best Sources: whole grains, legumes, sweet potatoes, cauliflower, broccoli and strawberries, liver, milk, fish and poultry

Pyridoxine (Vitamin B6)
RDA/DRI Under age 50: 1.3 mg (men and women)
      Over age 50: 1.7 mg (for men)
            1.5 mg (for women)
Supplement 50 mg per day (for men and women)

Toxicity Level: 200 mg long term use; 2,000 mgs/day can produce nerve damage.
Best Sources: liver, poultry, meat, fish, nuts and seeds, bananas, mangoes, prune juice, grapes, tomatoes, soy beans, Brussels sprouts, lima beans, brown rice, and wheat germ

Adequate vitamin B6 is important in carpal tunnel syndrome, depression, and diabetes (improved with 50-100 mgs/day supplement). A 50 mg supplement will reduce nausea of pregnancy, and help both osteoporosis and premenstrual syndrome.

Pyridoxine, together with B12 and folic acid, tend to reduce the blood's homocysteine levels, which protects against heart disease. Most of us get enough B6 and B12 each day from our diet. However, vegetarians may be lacking in both and may need to take supplements of both of these vitamins. Other people who need vitamin B6 are those who are minimizing their protein intake. Supplementing pyridoxine in allergy-based diets may also be called for. This is because protein (being restricted in the allergy diet) is the most common trigger for most allergies. Hence, an allergy diet may reduce protein enough to require B6 supplementation.

Cobalamin (Vitamin B12)

RDA/DRI   2.4 micrograms both sexes; Individuals aged
                51 and older should take a B12 supplement
Supplement 200 micrograms per day, both sexes

Treatment notes: 1000 micrograms orally, per day. Helps with AIDS, Alzheimer's disease, depression, diabetic neuropathy, low sperm counts, multiple sclerosis, and tinnitus (ringing in the ears).
Toxicity Level: 3,000 micrograms long term use.
Best Sources: found only in animal foods—liver, kidney, eggs, fish, cheese, meat. Rice and soy milk may have vitamin B12 added.

Vitamin B12 plays an important role in keeping blood healthy and in promoting healthy nerve function. Deficiency can cause chronic fatigue, constipation, depression, headaches, moodiness, and memory loss. Because vitamin B12 is found mainly in animal foods, vegetarians are at risk for deficiency. Vitamin B12 deficiency is frequently found in people as they age. This is because less stomach acid is produced. Stomach acid is needed for proper absorption of vitamin B12.[11] Therefore, supplements are routinely suggested for people over the age of 50.[12] As we age, we produce less stomach acid and so are less able to separate vitamin B12 from food.

Vitamin B12 is commonly considered for people with multiple sclerosis and other neurologic diseases. A deficiency in B12 and/or folic acid can lead to a set of symptoms or problems quite similar to those seen in MS.

Vitamin B12 can be taken orally but it's not well absorbed, and is also dependent on the acidity of the stomach. Suffice it to say some people will need supplementation. In many people this may need to be administered either under the skin (subcutaneously) or into the muscle.

Some people can take vitamin B12 under the tongue (sublingually). This method bypasses the liver and the breakdown that potentially happens to it there upon absorption. Though vitamin B12 is not well absorbed (worst case, only about 1.5% of an oral dose is absorbed), Dr. Michael Murray in the *Encyclopedia of Nutrtional Supplements* states that B12 taken orally works well.[13] The solution to its poor absorption, he says, is to take it in higher doses so that an adequate amount will be absorbed. A dose of 1,000 micrograms (1 mg) daily will solve the problem of this vitamin's poor absorption.

Vitamin B12 is now available in a second format—hydroxycobalamin (rather than cyanocobalamin). It has been suggested for a number of years, even by the American Medical Association, that hydroxycobalamin is a better choice. It can be requested from your pharmacist, who can obtain it directly in either of the above formats. It might be an important consideration for anyone with a neurologic illness.

The most common vitamins suggested to people with multiple sclerosis tend to be vitamin B12 and folic acid. It has been suggested that they may improve energy levels and reduce fatigue problems. In a lucky few, these vitamins may help or even reverse some neurologic symptoms.

Minerals

Calcium
RDA/DRI 1,000 mg (adults under 50 years of age)
1,200 mg (over 50 years of age)
Supplement approximately the RDA level

Toxicity Level: at least 2,500 mg
Best Sources: Dairy products, tofu (if made with a calcium-based coagulant), kale, spinach, broccoli, nuts, canned sardines with bones, molasses, cooked dried peas and beans

Calcium is confusing, as people are never sure which type to take. Some calciums are better absorbed, but the most important thing to know is that if you take vitamin D with calcium, you get up to 80% absorption. Normally, calcium absorption runs at about 20-30%. You can also increase calcium absorption from supplements by taking the supplement with a meal in doses of 500 mg or less.[14] At least a part of your calcium supplement, however, should be taken with vitamin D, and it should be taken at bedtime. Calcium has the side benefit of helping people sleep; it has been called "Nature's Tranquilizer".

If you have extra calcium and vitamin D working in your body through the night, you're going to have less likelihood of your body resorting to getting the calcium it needs from your bones. This means that you help prevent the removal of calcium from your bones. You also increase the length of time that the calcium can be laid down into your bones. This reduces the likelihood of developing osteoporosis.

In his book *Real Age,* Dr. Roizen says it is vitally important to prevent osteoporosis because it is the major cause of hip fractures and broken bones in the elderly. Once these fractures occur, the elderly begin a downhill spiral. Even though a person may immediately improve after such a fracture, more than 40% of patients require long-term nursing care. More than half the patients who have broken a hip never regain their former quality of life.

Calcium supplements containing bonemeal, dolomite, and/or oyster shells are best avoided. All of these can contain lead or other heavy metals that may be toxic. Calcium carbonate in particular is best taken with food; calcium citrate may be taken at any time, either by itself or with food. However, both can cause some constipation. If constipation is a problem, increase fiber by eating more fruits and vegetables each day.

Even if you are under age 30, you should be getting lots of calcium now. Up until age 35, the body tends to store calcium in the bones, and less calcium is lost from the bone. After age 35, the body tends to lose more calcium from bone than it conserves. This leads to a gradual loss of calcium from bones which in turn weakens the bone structure, leading to osteoporosis. Calcium the body stores in bones early in life becomes the surplus stores drawn upon later in life.

Calcium also has other special purposes in the body. It is used for nerve transmission and messaging between cells. It has also been shown to lower blood pressure. Taking calcium does not interfere with blood pressure medications or drugs used for chest pain (i.e., calcium channel-blocking drugs).

Remember that it's very important to take calcium with vitamin D. Also, we now believe that osteoarthritis—which was initially classified as a wear-and-tear disease, is actually autoimmune related. Vitamin D and calcium taken together can slow the progression of osteoarthritis and perhaps even prevent it. A large U.S. study[15] of arthritis patients showed that people with low levels of vitamin D and calcium had three times as much likelihood for rapid progression of their disease.

Magnesium

RDA/DRI 420 mg (for men) 320 mg (for women)
Supplement about 500 mg per day
Toxicity Level: 800-1,000 mg per day

Treatment notes: further increases beyond 1,000 mg per day should be done only under the advice of a health practitioner. *Best Sources:* tofu, legumes, seeds, nuts, whole grains and, yet again, green leafy vegetables.

Magnesium is very important inside our body's cells. Magnesium is critical in energy production, especially in the brain, heart, liver, and kidney. The majority of North Americans do not get the RDA. Why? Because most of us eat considerable amounts of processed foods. Food processing refines out most magnesium (just as it does potassium!). What to do—eat more whole foods!

For many of us, the optimum amount recommended means we will need to supplement. Magnesium is best taken in combination with calcium. Take the two at bedtime—500 mg of magnesium and about 1,000 mg of calcium, as stated above. Magnesium is very important for energy metabolism, which means it is required for muscle contraction, nerve impulses, and even for storing energy in cells.

Stress, sugar, alcohol, and phosphates (found in soft drinks and processed foods) all deplete our stores of magnesium and calcium. We lose magnesium in our sweat, so heavy exercise calls for supplementation as well.

A 10-year study was conducted with over 400 people who were at risk for heart disease. Those who ate a magnesium-rich diet and therefore had good levels of magnesium in their bodies, had fewer than half as many complications as those who did not. In addition, people with a magnesium-rich diet had lower death rates related to heart disease.

Both the elderly and women during their premenstrual time should take magnesium supplements. This will reduce heart disease, kidney stones, cancer, osteoporosis, diabetes, fatigue, PMS, and menstrual cramps. A good test for levels of magnesium is measuring its presence in red blood cells, as it is mostly an intracellular mineral (just like potassium).

Selenium

RDA/DRI   55 micrograms (men and women)
Supplement Highest daily intake considered safe is 400
micrograms, so don't use supplements over
200 micrograms.

Toxicity Level: Toxic at over 800 micrograms and can even
cause nerve damage
Best Sources: The simplest way to get this dose of selenium into
your diet is to eat one or two Brazil nuts per day. Other food
choices are dairy products, onions, grains, nuts, chicken,
meats, and seafood. Organic selenium is better absorbed than
sodium selenite. *Sodium selenite* is the straight mineral form of
selenium. We absorb selenium from foods much better than
the straight mineral form.

Benefits of selenium include blocking the damaging effects of
heavy metals like lead, mercury, aluminum, and cadmium. Also,
selenium supplements may help inflammatory problems such as
rheumatoid arthritis, multiple sclerosis, eczema, and psoriasis.
Selenium deficiency has been linked to heart disease and cancer.
It has also been associated with exhaustion, high cholesterol levels, infections, liver impairment, and sterility.

In a 1996 issue of the *Journal of the American Medical Association,*[16] 200 micrograms of selenium per day decreased risk by
half for each of three cancers—prostate, colon, and lung.

Selenium is known to be an important antioxidant, preventing the formation of free radicals. It is common in many foods;
however, many of us now get our foods from areas which have
selenium-poor soils. It's important to know where your food
comes from. People who live on the west coast of North
America, particularly British Columbia, Washington, and
Oregon state, need to be aware that most of the soils around
them are selenium-depleted. Europe has a similar problem, so
check it out, or supplement.

Iron
    RDA/DRI   10 mg (for men)   15 mg (for women)
    Supplement   no supplementation recommended

Treatment notes: only if indicated by blood tests

There are more diseases from too much iron than from not enough. The situation is very different for people regularly losing blood, such as women experiencing heavy menses. Children are also at risk for iron deficiency; however, most people consume adequate levels of iron from food.

Popeye used to teach us that large amounts of iron were available in spinach. In reality, spinach contains *phytates*, which limit how much iron is absorbed. This is an interesting and important consideration which has applications beyond iron and spinach. Phytates in cereal grains limit the absorption of vitamin D as well. That's one reason people who eat a lot of grain products are usually at least somewhat deficient in vitamin D.

Zinc
    RDA/DRI   15 mg (for men)   12 mg (for women)
    Supplement   to no more than 30 mg per day

Toxicity Level: toxic effects of zinc occur with prolonged intakes of 150 mg per day[17]
Best Sources: very common in animal products, shellfish, nuts, legumes, whole grains, and fortified cereals. However, the zinc in plant foods binds to phytic acid and is not absorbed by the body.

Zinc is an important antioxidant and enhances immune system function. Zinc is also important in maintaining optimal concentration of vitamin E in the blood. It is essential for vision, taste, and smell. Unless you're a vegetarian or on a special diet, you probably get enough from your food. Too much zinc interferes with copper absorption. Take no more than 30 mg per day.

Manganese
RDA/DRI   None established
Supplement   adequate at 2-5 mg for both sexes

Toxicity Level: greater than 30 mg per day. Toxicity from oral intake is highly unlikely.[18]
Treatment notes: 5 to 15 mgs per day is called for in people with epilepsy, diabetes, and sprains and strains.
Best Sources: Nuts, whole grains, wheat germ, oysters, and dark molasses.

Chromium
RDA/DRI   50 micrograms per day for both sexes
Supplement   200-500 micrograms per day

Toxicity Level: 1,000 micrograms per day
Treatment notes: 400 micrograms considerable benefit to losing body fat. Chromium's benefit in acne improvement is in the 400-500 micrograms per day range.
Best Sources: found readily in whole grains, meats, dairy products, and even beer.

We know that chromium is important for glucose metabolism and insulin secretion. It is particularly important in glucose metabolism in diabetics. The fine tuning of body cells' response to insulin may be how chromium can promote weight loss. A deficiency of this mineral can lead to fatigue and anxiety. In recent years, there's been talk that chromium extends your lifespan; however, the reality is that this conclusion is based mostly on animal studies and most have not been well-proven.

Too much chromium may result in uneven heartbeats, higher blood pressure, and problems with psychosis (mental instability). Trivalent chromium is very safe. There have been no significant side effects reported from chromium supplementation to date.

Potassium
RDA/DRI   1.9 to 5.6 grams per day

Treatment notes: for potassium depletion, usually via kidneys with fluid loss, and high blood pressure: 2.5 to 5.0 grams per day. If you are on digoxin, potassium-sparing diuretics, or ACE inhibitors, do not take potassium supplements. Check with your physician first.

Potassium first, and magnesium second, are the two most important minerals inside our cells. If we eat lots of fruits and vegetables, we should have adequate potassium intake.

Sodium
If we eat mainly processed foods, we probably get more sodium than we can possibly use or need. The minimum amount of sodium needed for good health is 116 mg a day; yet the average North American consumes more than 4,000 mg per day.

When you buy pre-packaged or canned foods, read the label. Some ingredients might not seem salty but actually contain large amounts of sodium. Examples would include cheese, preserved meats, and many condiments. Therefore, even if you cut back on table salt, it is usually the salt hidden inside processed foods that accounts for most of your sodium consumption. The only time to be concerned about taking in enough sodium is when you're doing very strenuous exercise on a hot day. Sodium depletion is usually only a concern for endurance athletes who have prolonged strenuous activity in a hot environment (e.g., marathon runners). A regular diet after exercise (i.e., without any extra salt added to it), will replenish any salt lost in physical activities.

Key Definitions
Free Radicals: A free radical is a very reactive molecule with spare electrons that can attack and destroy cells in our body. They

cause aging and trigger the three main killers—heart attack, cancer, and stroke.

Antioxidants protect us against free radical damage. Antioxidant nutrients include beta carotene, vitamins A, C, E, and selenium.

Natural Food Supplements

Alpha Lipoic Acid
    RDA/DRI   None established
    Supplement We recommend 120 mg per day

Toxicity Level: None established

Lack of information about Alpha lipoic acid is probably due to the very recent awareness of it. Do not confuse this with alpha-linolenic acid, which is an essential fatty acid.

Alpha lipoic acid is interesting because it is an antioxidant that is both water *and* fat soluble. As such, it can really help the recycling of other antioxidants and can boost *glutathione* levels (these are often very helpful in removing toxins from the body). It can also neutralize free radicals that can be a problem for us, particularly in glucose metabolism.

Acetyl-L-carnitine
    RDA/DRI   None established
    Supplement We recommend 500 mg per day

Toxicity Level: None established

Carnitine is getting more and more attention these days. It is very important for energy metabolism. Carnitine supplementation may improve the use of fat as an energy source.

Carnitine is the transport chemical that the body needs for moving fatty acids across membranes of cells into the energy factory—the mitochondria. Meat and dairy products are the major food sources. The redder the meat, the higher the carnitine.

Flavonoids (or Bioflavonoids)
RDA/DRI   None established
Supplement   We recommend 250 – 500 mg per day

Toxicity Level: None established

Flavonoids are beneficial phytochemicals, or chemicals produced by plants. You get only minute amounts of these if you eat a diet high in processed foods. If you eat a diet rich in a variety of fresh fruits and vegetables, you will get lots of phytochemicals.

The flavonoid most studied is *quercetin,* large amounts of which are in red grapes. Others include *proanthocyanin* and *anthocyanin.* Flavonoids are everywhere in nature. They are the pigments we see in fruits and vegetables—yellow in citrus fruits, red and blue in berries (like in blueberries). They're often present in the skins, peels, and outer layers of lemons, grapes, plums, grapefruit, and apricots as well. Eat a large number and variety of fruits and vegetables from as many different places as possible. Eat at least five servings per day, or up to 10 *or more* servings (1 serving = 1/2 cup or 125 ml or 1 medium fruit). Flavonoid supplements tend to be expensive, and in many cases won't be necessary if your diet is varied.

Flavonoids are critical to health and longevity. They are known to reduce inflammation and allergic reactions. They combat viruses and cancer-causing agents. In addition, they are powerful antioxidants and protect us from heart disease. Eat your way to health!

Isoflavones are a type of phytochemical usually present in soy products. They have an estrogen-like effect. This may be why they have been useful to inhibit things like prostate cancer in men and breast cancer development in women.

Lignins – These are present in flax seeds, and were alluded to in an earlier chapter. Flax seeds contain omega-3 fatty acids, which most of us are very short of. They also contain lignins. Lignins have been shown to lower the incidence of heart disease *independent of the omega-3 fatty acid effects*. In addition, lignins have been shown to be an excellent source of fiber, which reduces bowel cancer, enhances regularity, and lowers cholesterol.

Co-Enzyme Q10 (or Ubiquinone)
RDA/DRI   None established
Supplement   We recommend 100 mg/day. Best in soft gelatin capsules with Co-Q10 in an oil base

Toxicity Level: None established

Co-Q10 is a fat-soluble enzyme. Initial research involved heart problems, heart failure, and heart muscle conditions, especially in Japan. Co-Enzyme Q10 acts like a vitamin but, unlike a vitamin, can be manufactured in the body. It is particularly important for some of the energy factories inside the cells, and can be a very good antioxidant. Most of the research to date has been done in cardiac work ability, where it seems to offer a significant increase, i.e., it improves heart function and lowers blood pressure. Lower blood pressure usually reduces heart work.

Some data suggests Co-Q10 helps in gum (periodontal) disease, diabetes mellitus, preventing cancer, and enhancing immune function.

SAMe
RDA/DRI   None established
Supplement   We recommend 200-400 mg per day

Toxicity Level: None established
Treatment notes: Doses all start with 200-400 mg, but depression and osteoarthritis may call for four times this amount.

SAMe is the shorthand for S-adenosyl-L-methionine. It functions closely with folic acid and vitamin B12. SAMe is most often low in the elderly if they have depression, osteoarthritis or some liver disorders. It is suggested in these disorders, as well as in fibromyalgia and migraine headaches.

Glucosamine
    RDA/DRI   None established
    Supplement   500 mg/day

Treatment notes: see below; particularly helpful in osteoarthritis
Food Sources: None
    Glucosamine sulfate is the preferred form to use. It is needed to stimulate the key structural component of cartilage. Cartilage building and repair is essential for joint function. Hence, it can improve many arthritis problems. Glucosamine sulfate has better research behind it than cartilage extracts (including chondroitin). It outperformed ibuprofen in a study of 1,500 patients, for pain relief, after four weeks. Also NSAIDs such as Ibuprofen tend to slow cartilage healing and so may worsen joint problems. Source is chitin (hard shell of a shrimp, lobster, and crab).

Ambrotose^{TM} — "The Other Simple Sugars Needed by the body as Glycoproteins"
    RDA/DRI   None established
    Supplement   two capsules twice a day

Treatment notes: one to three teaspoons (5-15 mls) of Ambrotose powder per day
Toxicity: none reported; unlikely for a simple sugar in its clean form from plants; likely well over 100 teaspoons per day.
Food sources are fresh aloe vera, maple syrup (contains some mannose), fucose (present in some mushrooms). Other food sources are yet to be determined.
    Glycoproteins are combinations of simple sugars (like glucose in glucosamine) and simple proteins. Our body uses these

six other simple sugars to make glycoproteins that are important in cell-to-cell signalling and transfer of information.

These simple sugars are in the latest nutrition and biochemistry texts of today.[19,20] Some of the sugars are mannose, fucose, and n-acetyl-glucosamine (close relative of glucosamine).

Emu Oil Capsules
RDA/DRI   None established
Supplement   500 mg – 1,500 per day

Treatment notes: consider in inflammatory conditions such as arthritis, multiple sclerosis, inflammatory bowel disease, and psoriasis

Toxicity: None established, with thousands of years' experience
Data is limited to date, beyond the "Inflammopharmacology" paper of 1997. Personal reports include:
  i)   improved energy
  ii) improved blood sugar control in diabetes
  iii) lower cholesterol
  iv) less arthritis pain
  v)   less back pain

Dr. Bill Code:

> I take 2,500-3,000 mg per day. Morning is best for the energy boost emu oil capsules provide. Emu oil and other oils are better absorbed in the absence of calcium. Hence, I take my emu oil in the morning and calcium supplement at bedtime. I feel it helps me with my multiple sclerosis. My theory is that it reduces the likelihood of an acute episode—which starts as inflammation. In addition, emu oil is a collection of the many fat-soluble phytochemicals in this bird's diet. Emus are here after 80 million years as a species. That tells me something.

Fiber Supplements
    RDA/DRI   25-35 grams per day
    Supplement   start with 1-2 grams before meals; aiming
        for 35 grams per day

Treatment notes: start gradually and increase. Known to be useful in obesity, diabetes, kidney and gallstones, heart disease (lowers cholesterol and bad lipids), most bowel diseases, and even autoimmune disorders such as multiple sclerosis.
Best Food Sources: Virtually all whole fruits, legumes, vegetables, grains, and nuts.
    Beneficial effects of fiber, include:[21]
  a)   improved gut transition time (less constipation)
  b)   slows stomach emptying so reduces insulin spiking
  c)   increased feeling of fullness (satiety)
  d)   increased pancreas digestive enzyme secretion
  e)   increased stool weight
  f)   more advantageous intestinal bacteria
  g)   increased production of short-chain fatty acids (useful for energy)
  h)   decreased serum lipids (including cholesterol)
  i)   more soluble bile
    In summary, if in doubt, take more fiber. It reduces bowel diseases, including cancer, and prevents or helps treat obesity. Safety considerations—avoid fiber supplements in pill form if you have an esophagus disorder (e.g., troubles swallowing or esophageal stricture). Beyond that, fiber, fiber, fiber!

Essential Fatty Acids
    RDA/DRI   None established
    Supplement   Refer back to Chapter 1. We recommend
        1-2 tablespoons of flax oil per day.

    Toxicity Level: None established

70% of North Americans are deficient in the omega-3 essential fatty acids. They are particularly important in nerve generation, regrowth, recovery, and in the myelin covering around nerves. In addition, omega-3 fatty acids are vitally important for their ability to reduce blood clotting, and therefore may have a role in the long-term reduction of strokes and heart attacks.

Some Key Herbs

Be careful with certain herbs. Comfrey is known to cause liver damage, as are other herbs such as sassafras, chaparral, germander, and pokeroot.[22]

The Ginsengs – These are the most widely used and studied herbs. Panax (Chinese/Korean) ginseng's benefits include enhanced energy, improved recovery from exercise, better oxygen use during exercise, reduced exercise-induced lactic acid buildup. Particular attributes include improved listening and visual reaction times and improved vitality and well-being.

Echinacea should not be taken regularly or routinely. It is useful for boosting your body's natural immune system, but more particularly with respiratory or breathing-airway type infections. People allergic to plants in the sunflower family should avoid echinacea. Take echinacea only for a few weeks at a time when you get cold or flu symptoms.

Ginkgo biloba is from the Chinese ginkgo tree. It appears to increase blood flow in the brain as well as having antioxidant properties. It may help improve cognitive function in people with Alzheimer's disease or other forms of dementia. Fortunately, there are no known side effects to taking Ginkgo biloba. Therefore, it is certainly worth a try if you feel your thinking is not clear or your memory is not what it should be.

St. John's Wort has had some success in preventing or treating depression. It is also thought to have some anti-inflammatory abilities. Individuals taking anti-depressant medication must check with their physician before taking St. John's Wort.

Valerian is often used for stress reduction or relaxation. Although the source of the infamous Valium, it is itself not felt to be addicting.

Garlic – go organic. A powerful antioxidant and boost for the immune system.

Economy/Quality Supplements

1. Eat a varied, whole-food diet that is as organic as possible.
2. Grind and take two tablespoons of organic flax per day (less than $5/month).
3. Take 1,000 IU Vitamin D3/day for health in Canada (less than $2/month). If autoimmune diseases are present, take 4,000 IU Vitamin D3/day for treatment (less than $6/month)
4. Take a multivitamin/mineral supplement with a good spectrum:
   (a) if over 50 years of age, without iron
   (b) women of childbearing age, extra folic acid and iron
   (c) if over 50 years, 25 micrograms vitamin B12 per day
   (d) take calcium with vitamin D, especially at bedtime
   (e) selenium: 200 micrograms/day
   (f) vitamin E: if under 50, at least 400 IU/day; if over 50, consider 800 IU/day
   (g) vitamin C: 500-1000 mgs/day

Tips for Your Choice of Multivitamin/Mineral
1. Look for 100% of the RDA for seven vitamins (A, B1, B2,

B3, B6, B12, C). If over 50, look for 25 micrograms of B12 and 400 micrograms folic acid.

2. Get a minimum of minerals, particularly RDA of zinc, copper, and at least 25 micrograms chromium.
3. Add calcium (1000 mg) and selenium (200 micrograms) separately.
4. Avoid excesses, such as phosphorus (we all get enough from our food), B-6 (stop at 200 mg), beta carotene (stop at 15,000 IU), and iron.
5. In general, a good multivitamin/mineral and then top-ups in key personal areas such as vitamin D, calcium, selenium, flax seed, glucosamine, emu oil, and fiber.

CHAPTER 7

The Farmed Emu, its Agricultural History, and Oil Processing

The emu is the world's second largest bird. It is native to Australia and graces their nation's coat of arms. As a species, it is very old, and belongs to the family of flightless birds that includes the ostrich of Africa, the rhea of South America, the cassowary of northern Australia and Papau New Guinea, and the kiwi of New Zealand. The emu is a woodland bird of southwestern Australia. This is in contrast to the rhea and ostrich, which are desert birds.

Of all these birds, only the emu has a large fat pad on the back which stores nutrition. This fat pad is not unlike a camel's. In fact, the first part of *Dromais novae hollandidiae* (the Latin and scientific name for the bird) is short for *dromedary* (or camel). This is where the word or name *Dromais* originates.

The emu originated from the dinosaur. Research suggests that the emu has been on earth for some 80 million years. The Australian aborigines, who have long revered the bird for the medicinal qualities in its oil, tell a story of how the world was formed: An emu egg was thrown in the air and, upon breaking up, caused the world to be born.

The emu is one of the oldest living beings on the planet outside the ocean. It has a four-chambered heart and certain other developmental characteristics. By comparison, the ostrich is only some 50-60 million years old. In fact, an emu and ostrich are no more alike than an ostrich and a chicken.

The other things that make the emu quite similar to the dinosaur are its three toes—the two toes of the ostrich with one big one and one smaller one are more characteristic of a sub-set of dinosaurs which was less prevalent and less common. Another is the very tiny wings or front arms of the emu, being the size of just two of our fingers. In a bird that weighs in at 100 pounds and stands 6 feet high, this is very small. Compare that to the ostrich, which has wings much more like human arms than that of the tiny wings of the early dinosaurs. Today, we know many dinosaurs had air pockets in their bones. This is consistent with all birds existing today.

The emu's egg is dark green, and dinosaur eggs were also thought to be green. The dark green egg of the emu is quite unusual in today's world. Its color is due to the presence of *biliverdin*, part of the bile pathway in humans and other animals (*verde* meaning green). From the point of view of camouflage, this would make the eggs very hard to see in dark green grass. This is very important to the flightless emu, which lays its eggs on the ground. Once the female lays six to eight eggs, the male will sit on this clutch. He will sit for 52 days without eating, drinking, or defecating. His body temperature drops 2°C. Meanwhile, the female will lay 2-4 more eggs (one every three days) and the pair will move these in with the other eggs.

The female of this pair moves on to new relationships after 10-14 days. By spring, she will have two thirds of her chicks fertilized by males other than the first one. Only the emu and kiwi—a small nocturnal bird of New Zealand—preferentially lay in the winter. Emus eat very little all winter and primarily live off the fat pad they built up during spring, summer, and fall.

The male will hatch his chicks after 52 days. How he manages to hatch eggs laid up to a month apart, all in the space of

48 hours, is one of nature's mysteries. He will then parent and raise the chicks to 6-8 months of age. By now, they are 5-6 feet tall and ready to fend for themselves. The same or another female will chase the chicks away and the pair will start the process again.

Female emus are 10-15% larger than males. Females drum or boom with an air sac in the front of their neck. It is a deep, ancient sort of sound, not unlike a heartbeat. In the wild, emus tend to form social groups of twenty to forty birds. They will travel hundreds of miles in search of food and water. This unique bird has long been an important part of Australian aboriginal culture. The emu plays roles in their dances, stories, and namings of the dream time.

The aborigines used all parts of the bird—similar to the buffalo of the North American Plains' native. Today, we still use 95% of each bird. One bird yields 15-20 pounds of fat, 25 pounds of boneless meat, and 6-7 square feet of strong, supple, and finely stippled leather.

Emus are raised naturally on a mixture of grazing and grains. They have an excellent immune system so there is no need to use antibiotics or hormones in their growth. Chicks are hardy as well and adapt to most climates—including wet ones. Emus love the water. While they swim, they have their head and neck some two feet above the water's surface. It is unusual for us to have an animal with so many attributes that is also ecologically good for the planet. As usual, nature's wisdom is best.

Emu Oil Processing

The emu has a large fat pad across its back, as well as some internal fat. Best evidence to date relates that both of these sources exhibit the special characteristic actions of emu oil. An important part of processing is that the fat be recovered from the animal cleanly, whether this is done with liposuction or when the animal is processed for its meat, leather, and fat. Occasionally, people suggest that there is a difference between the two sexes as far as the usefulness of the fat is concerned. It's difficult to understand how this could be so. Emu fat produced into oil from birds 5 and 6 months of age seems to have the special properties we speak about. This is pre-puberty in the bird, with puberty not being reached until at least 10-15 months of age. Sometimes puberty occurs even later, depending on the birds' diets, stress levels, and other factors. With this understood, it would be very surprising to have a difference in a property of fat between the two sexes.

The other interesting thing about emus, is that both members (male and female) have high progesterone levels during the time of the breeding, laying, and hatching cycle. This is probably why the male does such a large degree of nesting.

Once the fat is removed from the animal, it is immediately frozen or processed. At this time, in North America and in Australia, virtually all of the fat is frozen—the sooner the better. It is characteristically frozen in block sizes of no more than 4-5 inches or 10-15 centimetres thick. It is best frozen with space all around it so that freezing can occur more rapidly. If it is frozen in chunks thicker than this, there is a risk of the inside of the fat going rancid, prior to its being frozen. The freezing slows down the speed of the enzymes that help break down the fat.

Another critical step is to minimize fat exposure to oxygen. This is accomplished either by vacuum packing, plastic application, or putting the fat into stainless steel containers. Carbon dioxide, carbon monoxide, or nitrous oxide should not be used because these molecules have a large amount of oxygen available for the peroxidation (or breakdown) process of fat.

The next step is to initiate rendering, which we typically call *processing*. In many ways it's similar to the rendering of lard from pigs and tallow from beef cattle. In Australia, the minimum amount rendered at one time is five tons (10,000 pounds). This is because rendering is done in only two major facilities in

Australia. These facilities must shut down from either lard or tallow to run through emu oil. In North America smaller processing units have been built. However, there is one—EPIC (The Emu Production International Co-Op), in Texas, which can process five tons per day. EPIC adapted its system from Texas A & M, rendering with steam-heat around jacketed stainless steel. The frozen fat is pressed by a hydraulic press against a machine that has a tearing-off or chipping action. The fat is then put into the pipeline system to be rendered and filtered away from its so-called "cracklings".

Frozen emu fat appears quite different compared to other animal fats, such as beef, sheep, pig, or even ostrich fat. The fat from these four species has lumps and occasional vessels. By comparison, emu fat is much more filled with blood vessels and connective tissue. This is probably due to the process of repeatedly taking fat on and taking fat off, each year—more like a camel. Experienced people can recognize emu fat just by looking at the outside surface of the fat. These become important issues because eventually, as emu oil is more and more in demand, people will try to slip in other fats to bring down the cost and, of course, try to get paid the same amount of money for it. Human ingenuity being what it is, someone will try it eventually. That's another reason why we've tried to develop a fingerprint or an indication of what an emu oil fatty acid analysis should look like. See our fatty acid analysis in the appendix at the back of the book.

In our initial facility, we took the frozen fat and cut it on a stainless steel bandsaw into small strips. Any stainless steel must be of a food processing standard quality. Next, a food grinder was used. Finally, it was put into an oven process. We initially used a laboratory-type oven and controlled the heat on it. The lower the heat, the less damage is done. Also, because the lower heat prolongs the time the rendering process takes, we reduce the oxygen flow over it as well. This allows the oil that drips down through a screen (a fairly fine mesh) to be reasonably clear and usually of very low peroxide. This reduces the need for deodorization (a final step in most oil processing).

Once the oil is strained, it needs to be filtered. The filtering is important for a couple of reasons. If the process is done carefully, there should be very little water left in the oil. That's very important. The filtering should also remove the majority of the proteins present in the fat. Proteins tend to be larger molecules, or they tend to be bound with other molecules. Some fat processing will precede the filtering by adding sodium hydroxide, which is a very potent base. It helps bind all the free fatty acids within the fat, but the concern is that it may strip some of the properties of the oil. Today, many people avoid that step. Instead, they filter the oil with a particular type of silica-based fine clay. This allows removal of the protein products and larger particulate matter. The fat is filtered down to 1 micron or even down to 0.2 microns. A filter of 0.2 microns will eliminate most of the bacteria within it. However, it will not eliminate viruses or fungal spores.

The above steps then produce a clear oil. Some people will take the oil at this point and then fractionate it further. This is done by letting it stand at a reasonably cool temperature so that the top component becomes relatively clear and the lower component becomes thick and creamy. If you then separate or decant these off from one another, you tend to get a product which is always clear at room temperature and the other (after this so-called winterization process) is usually thick and creamy at room temperature. Both of these are very temperature dependent. Actually, almost all of the fatty acid analysis done on one versus the other is very, very similar. From the fatty analysis profile, you virtually cannot tell which is which.

What this tells us is that both fractions have the same properties. There might be a slightly larger amount of polyunsaturated fats, because these tend to be in the clear fraction at room temperature, versus some that are slightly more saturated. However, testing of these does not seem to bear out this impression. Hence, it is more of a physical separation to please the consumer. This fractionation is very similar to the processing of cottonseed oil when it was first processed in the early 1900's. The top fraction, which was clear, was used for salad oil. This was the start-up of an ongoing concept of using a clear, almost odorless, light gold oil to consume with your salad. The lower fraction was of a more thick and creamy texture, which actually became the basis for many, many years of the Crisco trademark. Other oils, including coconut oil and palm oil, use a similar fractionation technique.

The final step in refining is deodorization of the oil. This is typically done with a burst of steam through the oil. How much steam has to be burst through it and how hot the oil must be is a function of how clean the oil is. Soybean oil can require a heat up to 550°C in an effort to deodorize it. This has the unhappy side effect of creating a large number of trans fatty acids. Emu oil can be deodorized at much lower temperatures. This is particularly the case if it is well looked after as a fat and in the rendering and filtering processes. Temperatures higher than 300°F should not be required. Each of these choices are important steps to consider in order to maintain the properties of emu oil.

Of course, centuries ago, emu oil was simply rendered in the sun. Sometimes, the Australian aborigines literally took a piece of fat and put it over the injured or bruised portion of the skin. It was tied on and only replaced as needed. The Australian sun can get to 140°F. Rendering the fat like this would secondarily result in a high peroxide value and an odor to it. Many people today would find this objectionable. Shelf life would be brief for the simple reason that the oil would continue to break down into peroxide and other free fatty acids over time.

It is the decision of the emu oil processor at the end of the rendering process whether to add an *antioxidant*, which slows the peroxidation process. There are a considerable number of these antioxidants, including BHA and BHT. Both of these are petrochemical products. Because BHA and BHT are artificial and sometimes irritating, they cannot be used by some people. Probably the majority of today's population, if asked, would prefer to have a naturally based antioxidant. The one that comes to mind most frequently is vitamin E. This is typically removed from vegetable oils and used as a by-product and sold independently of them. Unfortunately, a lot of these oils, particularly vitamin E oils, are extracted with hexane. You then get into another question of whether this is an ideal, natural benefit or not.

Alternative Methods of Oil Processing

Hexane works superbly well, and there is one patent which describes the use of hexane in extracting emu oil. It works very well, but the question is, have you managed to remove all the hexane once the extraction is completed? Hexane is very expensive and is recycled to be re-used. Therefore, it is prudent for the processor to try to recover all the hexane. However, it's important to think about this, particularly with emu oil, as it penetrates the skin so well. You have to worry about other agents present in the oil, as they will also absorb into the skin, along with the oil. If the agents are mildly toxic, neurotoxic, or carcinogenic, then they become important things to avoid. Today, approximately 95% of vegetable oils on our supermarket shelves are extracted with hexane.

Geographically-based Variances in Emu Oil

Canadian emu oil (or even that from southern Australia or the northern U.S.), is typically higher in alpha-linolenic acid than emu oil from warmer climates. We've seen numbers in the 3-5% range, and this number could easily be increased to the 20% range without too much difficulty by feeding flax or hemp to the animals. The interesting side note here is that oil that comes from animals or trees from colder areas is usually higher in the polyunsaturated component. If we think back to when we fractionated emu oil, it was felt there was probably more unsaturated components in the clear oil at the top. Why this functions the way it does is nature's solution for cooler climates. For example, cold water fish need a more liquid fat at the same temperature than if you took the same oil from warm water fish. Think of the more polyunsaturated as having an "anti-freeze" effect. The same happens in trees, in animals, and probably, to some degree in people. Emus raised in Canada have a double reason to have more polyunsaturated oils (the desirable ones). This includes both omega-3 and omega-6. Firstly, all of the plants raised in Canada—whether canola, hemp, or flax—are typically higher in omega-3 and omega-6 fatty acids too. Secondly, the animals in Canada live in a colder temperature and tend to have more of the polyunsaturated fats with more liquidity. So, they eat seeds and are fed diets that have the same advantages that the cooler climate has on them directly.

Dr. Bill Code

> I started to learn the dramatic effect of this when I attended the Oil Chemists' Society Meeting in 1997. I met a fellow who buys Canadian flax seed and sells it to American health food stores. He's obviously discovered that Canadian flax is unique, showing a higher level of the more healthy polyunsaturates. This will continue to be an important reason to use Canadian emu oil gel capsules. Also, gentle emu oil processing is needed to maintain these polyunsaturated fatty acids intact. Most Canadian emu oil has been processed gently and carefully, on a modest, non-industrial scale.

> As a follow-up to this, I wanted to test this hypothesis in emu oil. I am a member of the International

Standards Team for Emu Oil. Hence, I compared fatty acid analysis of emu oil from Canada, the U.S., and Australia. The Canadian emu oil was higher in both omega-3 and omega-6 polyunsaturated fatty acids. These are the desirable oils and essential fatty acids you learned about in Chapter 1. I presented this data at the 1999 American Oil Chemists' Society meeting. This was the third "Specialty Oils" session primarily on emu oil.

CHAPTER 8

Emu Oil & Skin Care

Our problems with the skin start early, right from our first experience with diaper rash, skin irritation, chicken pox, and so on. Some problems we see more acutely as we approach puberty—one of the first stages of aging. We'll discuss acne, pimples, and problems with skin changes, which include eczema and psoriasis. Our goal is to help with these issues and teach you how emu oil can help you with many of them, naturally.

Introduction

When we reach puberty, we may have a relative holiday with regard to skin aging concerns. But because we are so active at this time in our lives, there is the worry of outside sources of injury. These would include burns, sunburns, abrasions, irritations, dry and flaking skin, and assorted other skin problems that bother us through our 20's and early 30's.

By the time we are approaching our mid to late-30's, skin aging begins to be a concern for many people. Certain people are more dramatically affected by aging, particularly smokers and those who have very fair skin. Smoking aggravates the rate of skin aging and is actually one of the reasons why many plastic surgeons prefer not to, or will not, operate on people who are smokers unless they first quit.

Once we have reached this stage, we need to be aware of some of the changes that have happened in the body due to different nutritional needs. There are things you can put on your skin that either slow skin aging or to some degree may even reverse it. What you eat and how much water you drink go a long way to maintaining skin well-being.

From our late 30's to early 50's, we are at a time in our lives where, if a particular chronic illness is present, skin issues are more prominent. This would include illnesses such as diabetes, circulation problems, and other chronic health concerns such as alcoholism.

We tend to be in our 60's and 70's before we are finally becoming more relaxed about skin aging and aging in general. By this time, our skin is thinner, more fragile, and often demonstrates significant fine and deep wrinkles. Skin well-being is now even more dependent upon three things: nutrition, the things we put on it (creams and lotions), and the relative humidity of the air in our environment. In addition to this normal aging, there may be other problems such as skin ulcers (typically found on the lower legs of people in this age group), poor blood flow, pressure (bed) sores, and shingles (herpes zoster).

Part 1: Structure of the Skin

Your skin is one of the largest organs, covering your entire body. It provides you with a waterproof covering, and protects you from toxins, damage, and infection. It helps maintain body temperature and eliminates certain wastes. The skin is also the most sensitive organ, responding to the stimuli of touch, pressure, pain, and temperature. It repairs itself and is important in your body's production of vitamin D from ultraviolet sunlight.[1]

The skin is amazing. Do a little math and see how truly complex it is: one square inch (2.5 sq cm) of human skin contains:

- 650 sweat glands
- 65 hair follicles
- 234 feet of nerves
- 57 feet of capillaries

- 19,000 sensory cells
- 94 sebaceous glands
- 1,250 pain receptors
- 13 cold and 78 heat receptors

The Layers of Your Skin

The top layer is the *epidermis* (*epi* means outside and *dermis* means skin), which is made up of four sub-layers (only three where the skin is the thinnest). The stratum basale (bottom layer) is the base or germination layer. All the cells that will eventually be contained in the four layers are born here. When the cells are fully formed, they travel through all the layers on their way to the top layer where eventually they are sloughed off—a normal process.

The top or outside sub-layer is the *stratum corneum*—or fully keratinized (horny) layer. The cells of this layer are characterized by changes they undergo as they are pushed toward the surface.[2] The stratum corneum is the layer that is visible to us, the one primarily responsible for the look and feel of the skin. This is where healthy glow and youthfulness come from. Lymph cells, responsible for immunity, and melanocytes, which are responsible for skin color, are also in the corneum layer. These epidermal cells are formed in the germination layer.

The life cycle of skin cells is about 28 days—from formation to their movement to the corneum layer where they are finally shed. This life cycle extends to about 37 days after the age of 50. With psoriasis, this life cycle is reduced to 5-7 days in the affected area(s). Large amounts of water are held in the spaces between cells, and as we age, the skin's ability to retain this water is diminished *(see Figure 8-1)*.

The structural organization of the epidermis varies. For example, it is thickest on the palms of the hands and soles of the feet at 0.8-1.4 mm. In other regions, the epidermis is much thinner, averaging only 0.07-0.12 mm in most areas.

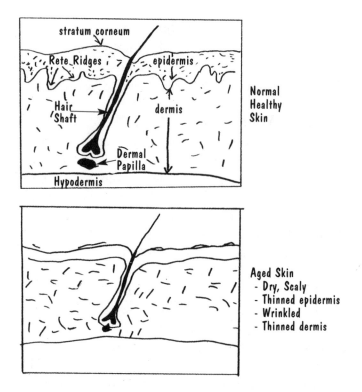

Figure 8-1: The major change that occurs in the lower layer of the skin is that approximately 20% of the dermal thickness is lost in elderly individuals. This may account for the paper-thin skin that the elderly develop.

Below the epidermis is the dermis, which binds the epidermis to the underlying tissues. The surface area between the two layers is usually uneven because it is the dermis which completely contains the "rete pegs". Rete pegs help give skin its tautness and elasticity. Think of a tent (your skin) being held up by stakes (the rete pegs). If the stakes are too short, or weak, the tent sags and wrinkles result.

Nerves always team up and travel with blood vessels, arteries, veins, and capillaries, and extend upward like fingers into the dermis, creating a wavy look when skin is viewed at a cross section *(see figure 8-2)*. The dermis is responsible for most of the structural support with its collagen and elastin protein fibers, and it is a network of these fibers that give the skin toughness and elasticity.

The dermis contains the capillaries and blood vessels which provide the skin with its nutrition. Also in the dermal layer are connective membranes, lymphatic vessels, nerve fibers, hair follicles, and sweat and oil (sebaceous) glands. Collagen is still, however, the main constituent. Collagen is made up chiefly of amino acids (proteins). It is collagen and its precursor procollagen which facilitate binding to water and maintaining the skin's high moisture content. The space between the collagen and elastin fibers is filled with *fibronectin* and *glycoproteins*, known as *glycosaminoglycans.*[3] *Mucopolysaccharides* (sugars) or *mucous-type* containing entities are a component of these *glycosaminoglycans.*

Sweat glands are found in the dermis and are part of the temperature regulating system. When sweat mixes with oily secretions, it forms a protective matte which is mildly acidic.

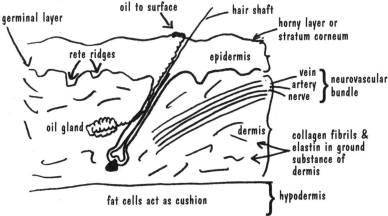

Figure 8-2 — Cross section of human skin showing "rete" ridges

The final, deepest layer of the skin is the *subcutaneous* layer (or hypodermis), consisting largely of loose and adipose (fat) tissue. These fat cells act as shock absorbers, protecting the blood vessels and nerve endings, and it is here where the muscle joins with the skin, and where the fibers and elastin bundles extend. The amount of adipose tissue in this layer varies greatly from one person to another—it is largely nutritional habits which will determine the amount of fat stored "under the skin". It also varies on every person from one region of the body to another. For example, there is usually a great deal of fat around the abdomen, as it is needed there to protect the organs, but is completely absent from the eyelids. The fat in the hypodermis also contains nutrients that are transported to the dermis and epidermis.

Eicosanoids and How They Affect Health

Omega-3 and omega-6 fatty acids (which are both present in emu oil) are converted in your body to hormone-like substances called *eicosanoids*. The parent fatty acids for eicosanoids are arachidonic acid (AA), from the omega-6 family, and eicosapentaenoic acid (EPA), from the omega-3 family (another reason why you *need* essential fatty acids). Obtaining fatty acids (such as those present in emu oil) from a natural source, where you have synergy working for you, may be the best way to get at least your partial daily allowance of essential fatty acids.

In the skin, the key eicosanoid produced from omega-3 fatty acids is PGI_3. Those produced from omega-6 fatty acids are PGE_2, leukotriene B_4 (LTB_4), and thromboxane$_2$ (TXA_2). They tend to work opposite to one another, but it has been found that many (though not all) of the omega-6-produced eicosanoids are what might be called *proinflammatory*. It is this action that is now seen as being responsible for many of today's health problems: asthma, allergies, arthritis, psoriasis, and other inflammatory diseases, perhaps even Alzheimer's disease.

Omega-3 fatty acids, by comparison, work opposite to those

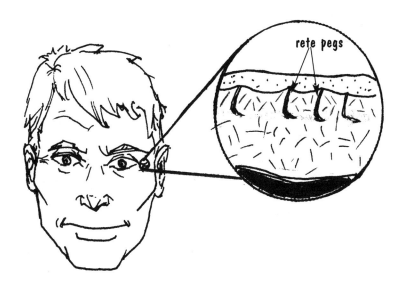

in omega-6. Do not misunderstand here: omega-6 fatty acids—especially in their pure, undamaged form—are vital to health. The key is to strive for the correct balance between the two.

Eicosanoids are fatty acids with oxygen attached. They are usually present in low concentrations, are chemically unstable, and have a lifespan of only a few seconds. Eicosanoids are found almost everywhere in the body and this includes the skin. Their production increases in response to a broad spectrum of biological effects. Many eicosanoids have competitive actions with one another. For example, PGI_2 *increases* blood flow in a tissue, while TXA_2 *decreases* blood flow in the same tissue. For simplicity, we'll focus on the three main eicosanoids involved in skin injury, healing, and recovery: PGI_2, leukotriene B_4, and thromboxane$_2$.

These key eicosanoids are derived or made from *20-carbon* essential fatty acids. You will remember these from our discussion of carbon chain lengths in fatty acid molecules—*eicosa* comes from the Greek meaning *20*. They are either taken in with food or synthesized from *18-carbon* essential fatty acid molecules: omega-3 (alpha-linolenic acid) and omega-6 (linoleic acid). (For review, you may want to go back and look at Figure 1-3.)

Most eicosanoids start from arachidonic acid, which is from the omega-6 pathway. However, the competitive eicosanoids (and in the case of skin, the "good" ones) are from EPA (eicosapentaenoic acid) of the omega-3 pathway.

Eicosanoids' effects include *contractility* (meaning, the size of the blood vessel and amount of blood flow) and *membrane permeability* (or degree of passing through the blood vessel or other cells). If skin is injured, for example, with a sunburn or dryness caused by exposure to the wind, one of the good eicosanoids to help speed healing would be PGI_2 (a *prostaglandin*). PGI_2 relaxes arterial *smooth muscle* and inhibits platelet aggregation (blood clotting).

Meanwhile, "bad" eicosanoids are also at work, the most common being TXA_2. TXA_2 contracts arterial smooth muscle and activates platelet aggregation (stickiness). This slows healing, generally speaking. Hence, PGI_2 and TXA_2 have opposite effects. Emu oil may act by increasing PGI_3 while either decreasing, or inhibiting, an increase in the production of PGI_2 and TXA_2.

Swelling in response to skin injury is usually filled with extra *collagen* and *fibroblasts* (i.e., connective tissue cells), thereby increasing scar size (*see figure 8-3*). Platelet aggregation is the start of scar formation and leaky membranes are the start of swelling. If emu oil can "fine tune" the body's own response, this may explain some of its speeding of healing and anti-inflammatory ability. (See discussions about the Snowden and Whitehouse article and the Lopez, et al article in the Scientific Studies appendix.) In this example, fine tuning of the healing process by emu oil permits quicker skin recovery with less scarring. See our summary of "Wound Healing" by M. Politis and M.F. Holick in the Scientific Studies appendix.

Also, a slow-releasing substance of *anaphylaxis*, which tends to increase swelling and which is now recognized as an eicosanoid (TXA₂), is blocked by the good eicosanoids present in emu oil. Unfortunately, the swelling, besides being uncomfortable, also reduces—sometimes drastically—the blood supply to the epidermis, which results in slowed healing. This is due to the fact that the bringing in of new raw materials and the taking away of infected or problem skin cells, is compromised due to the swelling.

There is an enzyme in the human body called *delta-5-desaturase*. This enzyme converts fatty acids taken in with food to

Injury to Skin & Healing

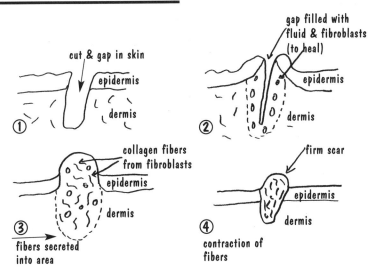

Figure 8-3 —1 through 4 demonstrate steps in normal skin healing. The result is a scar, keloid of firm tissue that will last forever. It may fade over two years. Emu oil minimizes the scar and speeds healing by fine-tuning the body's response. Hence, there is less overshoot or excess response.

"bad" eicosanoids. The *skin* lacks this enzyme, however. This is important: it means that the fatty acids in the emu oil cannot be converted into bad eicosanoids when applied to the skin. This is why emu oil on the skin has such a dramatic effect. More distinctly, pain is primarily due to the production of leukotriene-B_4 (a bad eicosanoid) and by blocking the production of this with the benefit of the good eicosanoids, it has the effect of rapidly reducing pain. This could be a good explanation of emu oil's effect on Herpes infections.

Using Emu Oil for Problems of the Skin

Herpes
Herpes is caused by the herpes simplex virus. One way it shows up is as a canker or cold sores. Emu oil not only takes the pain of herpes sores away very rapidly but also speeds healing. In fact, when the virus is starting up (people talk about that tingling sensation they feel, and they *know* it's coming), apply the emu oil lip balm mixture right away. The emu oil lip balm is preferable to the straight emu oil in the case of sores in and around the mouth because it contains beeswax, which tends to hold it on the skin. Without the beeswax, emu oil is absorbed so rapidly that you'll need to keep reapplying.

If the herpes sore is away from the nose or mouth, apply straight emu oil and put a band aid over top so that the area is literally bathed in emu oil for a 12 to 24-hour period. Start with the emu oil almost immediately. If you wait 24 or 48 hours, as some health experts have recommended, you will likely have more swelling and in general a longer road to healing.

When we get our first primary herpes virus as a child, it's usually all through the mouth. Children don't want to eat or drink anything because the pain is so bad. To give your child some relief, put some emu oil directly into the child's mouth, have him swish it around, and then spit it out. This will provide comfort for an hour or two and hopefully speed up healing. Emu oil is safe even if swallowed, so "no worries" on that score.

After that primary herpes infection, the virus rests quietly in the nerve pathways supplying the face and mouth. When our immune system is not functioning optimally due either to fatigue, poor diet, or excess stress, the herpes comes out of hiding and flares up with an outbreak on the skin. This is why herpes continues to recur whenever the immune system is not in top form. Why emu oil works so well is uncertain, but it probably has something to do with suppressing the body's inflammatory response—that is, it is working as an anti-inflammatory. In essence, emu oil fine tunes healing.

The discussion of herpes in this chapter has so far been limited to the Simplex No. 1 variety, which primarily appears on the face. The other variety—Herpes Simplex No. 2—primarily appears in the genital/anal region. In emu oil, we have something that will help either one.

Genital herpes is a sexually transmitted disease with very few treatment options. Outbreaks are very painful. Genital herpes is a risk factor for babies because they can be infected on their way through the birth canal. Hence, it is one of the indications for cesarean section even today. Emu oil, when applied to the site, will shorten the time frame of healing and reduce the pain involved. Genital herpes doesn't typically respond to oral medication because some of the virus components remain dormant in nerve cells. Therefore, even virus killing agents *(virucidals)* are often ineffective.

Other Common Skin Problems

Even when everything else fails, bed sores or leg ulcers will start to heal when emu oil is applied. Some research shows that if you take the essential fatty acids—omega-3 and omega-6—and put them on a wound, it will show improvement. The essential fatty acids in emu oil may account for its effectiveness in such cases.

It's not just fine-tuning the body's inflammatory response, but it is also supplying nutrition to the site. We know it absorbs well. We know that the fatty acids are very important for cell growth and division and recovery. Perhaps this is another way of providing the much needed nutrition to speed healing—put it right on the skin. The other way would be orally (with emu oil capsules), which also works well.

A veterinarian we know doesn't put the emu oil on right after surgery. However, she finds that if she administers capsules orally, the surgical sites heal more efficiently, there is less pain, and healing is enhanced. Again, it may be the fine-tuning of the inflammatory response, but the actual required nutrition is possibly also reaching the site.

Topically, emu oil is great on sunburns, and in fact works very well on any kind of burn. Data shows that it reduces scarring, speeds healing, and sufferers need fewer pain killers. Controlled trials conducted at Texas Tech were performed in the following way. Photos were taken of burn sufferers and compared by observers who were not told whether patients had emu oil, mineral oil, or corn oil applied to their wounds. First of all, patients recovered faster and used less pain medication with the emu oil and had less scarring. Also, and this is important: the patients preferred the emu oil.[4]

Keloids are bumpy skin growths on a wound (like proud flesh on a horse) and are an over-response to healing. In people prone to keloids or to an adverse reaction to sutures used for stitching, emu oil may reduce swelling and inflammation. In the same way, emu oil also helps acne. You tell most people to put emu oil on acne, and they don't see how it can help. They've always tried to get oil *off* their acne. But emu oil settles the acne down by reducing the swelling and inflammation. Irritation happens less, resulting in a smooth face again. It is important to know that emu oil is *non-comedogenic*, i.e., it doesn't clog pores, nor does it cause pimples or blackheads.

Primary Care of the Lips, Mouth, and Throat

We all care about how we look, that's why ladies wear lipstick or use lip balm. Men use lip balm too, especially those living in drier climates. We want to be comfortable and we want to look good. Chapped lips are no fun. But have you ever considered what is *in* the stuff you are putting on your lips? Years ago lipsticks in health food stores might have invoked a response like: isn't this is a bit extreme … after all, what harm could lipstick or lip balm do? The slick advertising of the large cosmetic companies draws us in again and again, but beware: there are ingredients in these products you want to stay away from.

Many lip balms today contain mineral oil. This is fascinating in that mineral oil is actually a mild skin irritant and, over time, causes more and more irritation of the skin. It's a clever marketing angle when you think about it: have someone apply lip balm because their lips feel dry, and 20 to 30 minutes later need to apply more because now they have a mild irritation problem to solve (and they also still have dry lips, most likely). Instead, the benefits of putting on an emu oil-based product are many—it will permit deep penetration to help the skin recover and won't cause any skin irritation—few products feel better.

Many people do not wish to put petrochemical products on their skin, recognizing that some of it is absorbed—and who could blame them? Over the years, we haven't had a lot of options, though. For decades, we've been using petroleum jelly, which is to some degree absorbed by the body. While it may not seem like much (a little lipstick or lip balm), it is the *cumulative* effect that we can't be certain of. And it isn't just the petrochemical ingredients. There are other ingredients that manufacturers use—not just in the manufacture of lip balms and lipsticks—but in all sorts of personal care products like shampoos, moisturizers, foundations, hand creams, body rubs, sunscreens, and so on. On page 215, you'll find a listing of common chemical constituents of popular drugstore and supermarket personal care products. You'll be shocked at the damage being done to your skin and, by extension, your body!

Justifiably, we are becoming increasingly concerned about what degree of these chemicals—petroleum-based and otherwise—is absorbed. Here's an important point: the inside of the lip, all of the mouth, and upper parts of the nostrils and breathing system have only one protective layer of skin cells. This is unlike other surfaces such as the face and hands and the rest of the body, where there are several layers of skin, providing a more resilient resistance to absorption. Obviously, most people would prefer a product that doesn't have any undesirable side effects, if absorbed. Emu oil is so much better: it can be combined with thickening agents such as healthy, non-toxic beeswax, which will also facilitate the body's recovery process and does so safely.

By the way, do you know what they use to make lipstick shiny? It's aluminum! Many of us have changed our pots and pans over the years because we fear that intake of excess aluminum will cause long-term memory troubles. However, many women use lipstick several times a day, not knowing that it contains a substance that in excess has proven to be toxic to the human body.

On the inside of the mouth, we may have recurring problems such as mouth ulcers or canker sores, and also general irritation along the gum line and inside the mouth. A good example would be gum irritations at the base of our teeth—gingivitis. Apply emu oil (yes, even inside the mouth as you heard about earlier with a child's herpes simplex) and it will greatly speed the body's healing, reduce discomfort or pain, and allow things to get back to normal more quickly.

Applying emu oil on the inside of the mouth is particularly useful for people who are undergoing therapy such as chemotherapy or radiation. These types of therapies, by their very nature, cause cell breakdown and death of rapidly dividing cells. The cells that line the inside of the mouth and stomach, in par-

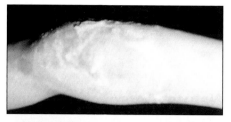

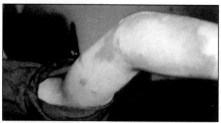

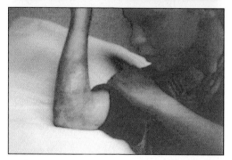

Gasoline Burn
(per gasoline ignition):
Emu oil was started
when he saw his
physician. He healed
rapidly and needed
very little of the pain
medication prescribed
to him.

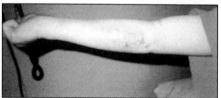

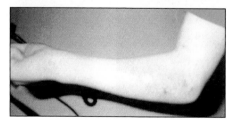

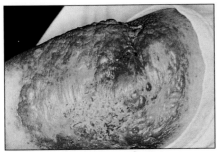

1

Sun "Poisoning":
*Severe sunburn and/or
reactions, results in 2nd
degree burns and blisters.
Rapid pain relief and
healing within two weeks
using emu oil.*

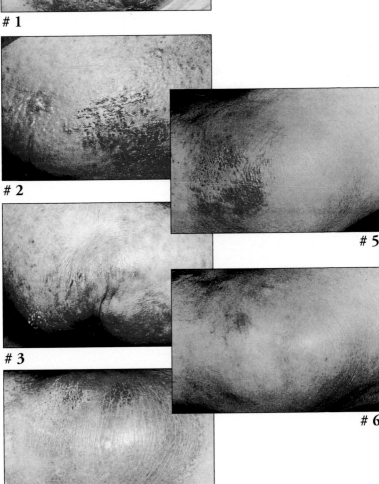

2

5

3

6

4

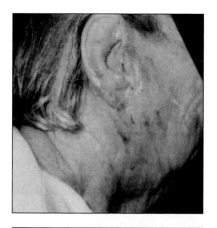

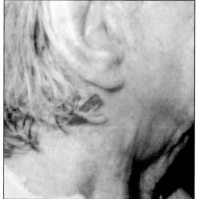

Eczema, elderly woman:
*Eight weeks of regular
(cortisone) creams brought
no success. Emu oil begun
and much improved at one
week, well healed by three
weeks.*

*See discussion of eczema in
Chapters 3 & 7.*

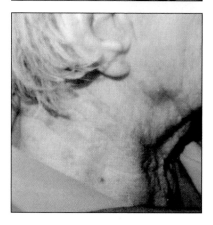

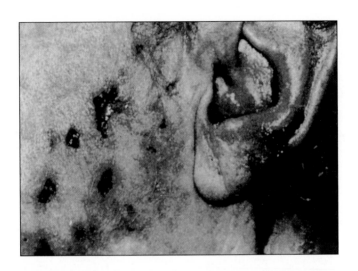

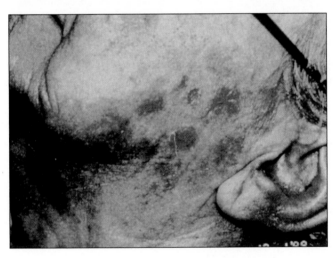

Herpes Zoster: *Prominent case of Shingles on the face, including left ear. Blisters are now deep ulcers. 2nd picture one week later, with only emu oil applied.*

See discussion of emu oil and Herpes Zoster in Chapters 3 & 7.

ticular, are some of the body's most rapidly dividing and multi-plying cells. They are killed off as a consequence of chemother-apy or radiation, which is trying to kill off the rapidly dividing cancer cells. This unhappy side effect can be minimized by applying emu oil in liquid form—just swish it around the mouth and spit or swallow. This very helpful, gentle, and inex-pensive treatment will help the body recover more quickly. It is amazing how much relief people get just from biting on a cou-ple of emu oil capsules every few hours as necessary. What we see with emu oil is ongoing improvement and enhanced quality of life even during one of the tough side-effects of this particu-lar type of cancer treatment. Radiation burns on the skin surface respond very well to emu oil, too.

Herpes Zoster
This is the virus chicken pox, or *varicella*. It typically affects chil-dren, and there is now a vaccine for it, but the vaccine isn't commonly used yet. Many people plan to expose their young-sters to chicken pox at an early stage because the older you are when you get it, the sicker you can become with it.

The main problem with chicken pox in children is the itch-ing and scratching. As much as you might tell a child not to scratch, they are unable to stop. Even if they manage not to scratch when awake, they will do it in their sleep. Typically, they've had antihistamine creams applied. Emu oil is particular-ly useful at blocking the itching and reducing pain and scratch-ing. It is the scratching and subsequent breaking of skin which causes the scarring later on, so emu oil may dramatically reduce this problem.

After the first infection with chicken pox (or herpes zoster), the virus remains dormant in the nerves over a long period of time. Therefore, it can recur later in life. It was believed that only the elderly or the sick (immune-suppressed) were vulnerable; however, we now recognize herpes zoster can happen in a large number of people, even at a younger age, and particularly when they're stressed and their immune system isn't working well.

When herpes zoster (also called *shingles*) strikes adults, some of the more common areas it affects is on either side of the body, coming around to the breast area in this T-5 or *thoracic-5* distribution *(see figure 8-4)*, and covering the nipple area and the entire breast. Herpes zoster also commonly appears on the face,

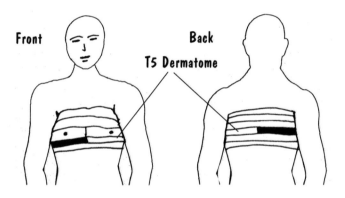

Figure 8-4: T5 is the most common "Shingles" distribution, i.e., the Thoracic 5th Nerve

involving the eye and the tissues around one eye. This is very painful and can cause blindness. Occasionally shingles happens in the groin or other regions of the body.

Shingles pain is very uncomfortable and very unpleasant. Unfortunately, the body tends to take the pain message and make it into a *recurring* message. This message recurs so often that it literally imprints on the brain and spinal cord. The result is that the pain persists even after the blisters and *vesicles* are healed. Any trigger that irritates that area (even seemingly benign items such as clothing or a gentle touch) often causes the imprinted pain message (wind-up) to return.

The pain is severe: a modest proportion of sufferers go on to suicide, feeling it is their only escape. The pain is intermittent and responds very poorly to opiates or narcotics. There hasn't been a satisfactory treatment yet. One treatment that has its roots in anaesthesiology is "nerve blocking" the pain over several days, usually for at least three days or three treatments. However, if this treatment isn't performed within the first three or four weeks of the pain, then the pain can be there for a lifetime.

We've seen a large number of cases—over 20—respond very well with the application of emu oil every 2-3 hours. It tends to take away the burning and irritation, enhance the rate of healing and, more importantly, seems to dramatically prevent the likelihood of developing the pain long-term; yet it is a completely non-invasive treatment.

Emu Oil and Cosmetics

If you're going to put something onto your skin—like acne medication or moisturizer—and expect it to have some therapeutic benefit, you expect it to be absorbed. After all, if it just sits on top, it really can't do any good, can it? By the same token, lipstick, as we've discussed, and products such as foundations, are also absorbed by your skin to some degree. It is prudent to understand first of all what the ingredients are, and secondly, what they are doing to your skin. They could be making you look older; they could be irritating your skin. Some products give you a healthy glow (that is, redness) by causing a mild inflammatory response. Some clog pores, not allowing your skin to breathe *(see Cosmetic Chemicals Table on page 215)*.

When you start to look at some of these issues, they can cause some concern. Now, look at emu oil as a base for cosmetic or skin products. Emu oil is a natural oil containing essential fatty acids and works as a natural anti-inflammatory. It works as an emollient, has anti-aging properties, and heals skin faster than most commercial skin products. Now, to explain all this.

What Emu Oil Can do for Your Skin

In the discussion earlier about eicosanoids, we alluded partly to what emu oil might do for the skin. The *chemical structure* or *molecular makeup* of emu oil is recognized as being very close to human skin. Emu oil is quite high in oleic acid, which is also reasonably high in human skin (though not as high as emu oil). The fatty acid composition of emu oil is also reasonably similar to that of human skin.

Emu oil contains a small amount of phosphorous, and this may also make a difference in how well it penetrates human skin. Emu oil, like many oils, is relatively non-polar (not electrically charged). A non-polar compound can travel through a cell much better than a polar compound, as a polar compound is positively or negatively charged and is usually stopped at the entrance gate to the cell. Whether a compound is polar or non-polar makes a big difference in its ability to move between cells.

Emu oil is a source of nutrients to the skin. Here's how it works. The skin has blood vessels supplying it with the nutrients it needs for elasticity, hydration, and healing. If there's injury such as bruising, a release of eicosanoids occurs, along with other responses, that cause swelling and edema (fluid accumulation). If you visualize this, you can imagine that the skin's surface—with this swelling—is now further from the blood supply. Your skin now has fewer white blood cells and nutrients reaching it and slowed removal of waste. The result is delayed and slowed healing.

So, in emu oil, we have a substance that supplies nutrients directly to the skin and penetrates the skin very well. What this suggests is that emu oil may help the skin heal (recover from injury) more quickly. It also tells us that emu oil has an anti-aging component due to improved cell function, cell change-over, and cell renewal—all things that tend to work against aging. Hollick's article (find sections of this article in the "Scientific Studies" appendix) states a 30% increase in skin

Cosmetic Chemicals Causing Adverse Effects
(more than contact dermatitis)

(alphabetical, from a list of more than 100)

Chemical	Effects
Coal tar derivatives	acne; carcinogenic
Lanolin (sheep oil)	acne; compounds of manufacturing process, e.g., ethylene oxide or dioxane are both potent toxins; 7% of people allergic
Mercuric compounds	heavy metal toxicity
Mineral Oil	contains benzo-a-pyrene and benzo-b-fluroanthene, both of which are carcinogenic
Nitrosamines, benzenes, toluene, dioxane, diethylene dioxide & phenylenediamines	all are carcinogens
Petrolatum (petroleum jelly) & paraffin	are carcinogenic
Propylene glycol	causes acne & dermatitis
Triethanolamines (TEAs) - a popular emulsifier	carcinogenic
Urea	prominent to severe contact dermatitis

thickness and enhanced tethering (reduces wrinkles).

Some scientists now estimate we have the genetic capability of living to 120 or 140 years—being useful, functional, and clear-thinking for that whole time. In order for this to be possible, however, we need to look extensively at our nutrition. Fatty acid optimization and nutrition—whether applied to the skin in the case of emu oil or whether taken internally in the way of omega-3 and omega-6 fatty acids—is key to skin healing.

The layers of every single cell in the body is a bilipid layer with some protein content in the middle. Best to think of it as sort of a fat layer on each side, like a sandwich, with some protein or *hydrophobic* (water hating) elements on the inside. Through this is a series of proteins, sometimes running crossways and sometimes going through the actual bilipid sandwich layer. These become channels and transmission sites for cell minerals, nutrients, and other substances.

Is Emu Oil an Emollient?

An *emollient* is a substance that softens tissues, especially skin and mucous membranes. Emu oil is an excellent emollient—it mixes well with skin tissues to soften them—and is a fair *emulsifier*. To *emulsify* is to mix a liquid into another liquid, making a suspension that has globules of fat (e.g., water and oil, shaken, is an emulsion).

A common emollient used in commercial skin care products is *potassium hydroxide* which, unfortunately, can cause irritation and is corrosive if ingested, causing pain, bleeding, and even death. In animals, tumours resulted when moderate amounts of potassium hydroxide were applied to the skin of mice. Obviously it is a good thing to avoid. It's used as an emulsifier in hand creams, as well as a cuticle softener and is extremely corrosive and may cause irritation of the skin.

Esters are emulsifiers and essential stabilizers found in creams and lotions. They give the lotions a less oily, more satiny or slippery (emollient) feel. Esters are the end-product of mixing fatty alcohols with acids. An easy way to spot an ester in your product is by looking for ingredients where the first word ends in "yl" (fatty alcohol) and the second word ends in "ate" (a fatty acid) such as *isopropyl palmitate.*

The presence of vitamin E oil or grape seed extract (both used as antioxidants) may cause problems. The reason is that these oils are most often extracted with hexane, and a topical reaction to this chemical is quite common. The other really important thing to remember is that makeup of all kinds becomes infected with fungus or bacteria as it sits in your bathroom. Your cosmetics should really be stored in the fridge. You can introduce bacteria and fungus into your products simply by using them on a regular basis. As mentioned before, proteins and water are great mediums for growing stuff—any kind of stuff (bacteria and fungi included) and water is the number one ingredient of most cosmetic products. That's why in straight oils or straight honey, you get almost zero growth, because bacteria and fungi need water and protein. Collagen, present in most cosmetic products, provides the protein required for bacterial growth. Hence, a product like emu oil, without water or protein, will keep longer. In fact, many "reactions" to cosmetics are due to secondary "bugs" or infectious bacteria growing in a product that has been opened, and that sits on your vanity for weeks at a time.

Ingredients derived solely from petroleum include mineral oil, paraffin, isopropyl alcohol, microcrystalline wax, and carbomers. Ingredients that are partially petroleum based will include syllables such as "ethyl," "methyl," "butyl," "propyl," "octyl," "PVP," "ene," and "eth." Ingredients such as *stearic acid* and *glycosaminoglycans*, or, commonly, those containing "stear-" and "gly-" in their names, add a rich feeling to the product. If you look at the profile of most animal fats, including emu oil, they contain some stearic acid (you will remember from the chapter on fats that stearic acid is simply a saturated fatty acid).

Ingredients starting with the letters "coc," "laur," or "myr," indicates a coconut source. Coconut oil has long been used as an emulsifier in many cosmetic products. It is a highly beneficial component of emu oil soap. A substance close to being an emulsifier is a *phospholipid*. Phospholipid molecules are one part *hydrophylic* (attracted to water) and two parts *lipophylic* (attracted to lipid substances)—very similar to an emulsifier. This is of course fairly close to the cell membranes that are held throughout the body. Let's not forget that the skin (being such a large organ) has the most to gain or lose by changes in your fatty acid intake. Remember, "intake" applies to both what we eat and what we apply to the skin.

The reason for this is simple: if you replace unhealthy or trans fatty acids with healthy fatty acids, the result is a more resilient and flexible cell wall, which will have more of a "soft" non-aging or anti-aging component to it. It might be best to think of *trans* fatty acids as being quite flat, almost like a straight line, whereas a *cis* fatty acid tends to be bent in shape, like a hockey stick or a corkscrew *(see figures 1-5 and 1-7)*. The curved or bent shape offers resilience and ideal shaping in the outside cell wall membrane. It may sound like a small thing, but when your trillions of skin cells have fluid and flexible outer walls, it can make a profound difference to your appearance.

Common Emulsifiers

Alkoxylated alcohols, alkoxylated amides, alkoxylated amines, alkoxylated carboxylic (fatty) acids, and *fatty alcohols* are all in a product to hold the oil-based and water-based ingredients together so they don't separate in the finished product. Of course, in the manufacture of creams and hand lotions, products that separate on store shelves or in your bathroom are not in very high demand. In the blending of emu oil products, the tendency is to stay away from emulsifiers.

It is often water that causes the problems in many of today's products. Water attracts bacteria and is a great growth medium for that bacteria. If you stay away from water, then you have a product that stays together regardless—you don't need extra ingredients that bind the water-based ingredients (because there aren't any) to the oil-based ingredients. Since emulsifiers are usually of an unhappy origin (as we've talked about above), you also have the advantage of having a product which will work better in the long term and will not have any toxic components to it.

You can weed out about 95% of potentially irritating skin care ingredients simply by looking for and avoiding certain substances. The number one substance and easiest to identify is synthetic fragrance. Look for products that use herbal extracts or essential oils to scent their products; avoid ones that list fragrance on the label as they contain synthetic hydrocarbons.

The second thing to avoid are color additives. Choose instead products that are colored by natural colorings or by the natural hues of the herbal extracts they contain. Avoid any product that uses FD&C or D&C colors. Finally, avoid petroleum derived ingredients. Instead, look for products that contain natural ingredients such as shea butter, beeswax, phospholipids, or hydrolized protein. Other acceptable ingredients are those with so-called large molecular weight *polymers*. These are listed as dimethicone, dimethicone copolyol, and cyclomethicone.

Can we believe that the chemicals in commercially prepared products are good—or at least not bad—for our skin? Do the manufacturers of these synthetics strive to create skin care products that closely imitate the protectant layer of the skin, thereby helping it retain its natural moisture content? This is debatable, and certainly part of the reason information provided in this book is so important. Everything large skin care and cosmetic companies tell you (and choose not to tell you) in their multi-million dollar television commercials and glossy magazine ads, shouldn't be taken at face value (no pun intended).

At the other end of the spectrum, we have natural manufacturers who promote their products as being therapeutic—nour-
ishing, healing, restorative, or otherwise providing some
improvement of various skin functions. However, there is a third
(rare) category of skin care manufacturing that goes well beyond
these two. This is a *cosmeceutical.* This is where skin and science
meet. Emu oil can best be classified as such.

Given all the undesirable ingredients out there, using emu oil
is very reassuring because it is a *natural* substance that is very
close in composition to the makeup of our own skin. It is highly absorbable, anti-aging, anti-inflammatory, and will not cause
any irritation.

CHAPTER 9

Emu Oil & Arthritis, Massage Therapy and Chiropractic

Arthritis by definition is *inflammation (itis)* of the *joint (arth)*. Inflammation, a painful product of arthritis, has four components—redness, pain, swelling, and loss of function. A simple example of inflammation would be a sprained thumb, which would be swollen, red, painful, and difficult or impossible to use.

We don't know exactly why emu oil works so well with inflammatory skin conditions, but whatever the process by which this works, the same process may be at work in the relief of inflammation caused by arthritis. In the last chapter, we told you the effect certain eicosanoids have on the skin. It is possible that the essential fatty acids present in emu oil produce eicosanoids that are beneficial to the skin. These eicosanoids and other substances in the emu oil then penetrate deep enough, working their way into the bloodstream. While we cannot be sure of this process, we do know that emu oil can be applied to one part of the body, where it is absorbed, relieving inflammation in another part of the body. In the Scientific Studies appendix, you will read about the Whitehouse and Snowden study, in which it was found that an animal with a sore *foot* experienced relief when emu oil was rubbed on its *back*.

Emu oil on its own can often help even those joints deep inside the body to a greater degree than one would anticipate. Typically it's very difficult to get relief of stiffness and soreness in a joint from just applying something to the skin. This is particularly the case with knees and shoulders. However, emu oil continues to surprise and impress by its ability to work on shoulders and knees. It can be applied "plain"—without any other ingredients added to it. If that isn't enough, it is combined with wintergreen (methyl salicylate), eucalyptus oil (which is also an anti-inflammatory, although to a lesser degree), and other things that may help penetration, such as isopropyl alcohol.

Sometimes emu oil has a "warming" agent added to it—typically camphor. Another ingredient commonly added is menthol, which has a cooling effect. Occasionally, people add menthol because it soothes the itch and irritation that results from isopropyl alcohol on the skin's surface. Many people avoid isopropyl alcohol, preferring to use something more naturally based than an alcohol derivative.

A number of studies have been done to date, and there have been some initial trials on humans. The study by Australians Drs. Whitehouse and Ghosh[1] was conducted to see whether the painful swelling that takes place in joints and bones would improve, and secondarily whether emu oil limits arthritis pain for people in either bone, cartilage, or swollen joints. Each of these clinicians have had over 25 years experience and published extensively on the evaluation and development of drugs used for arthritis.

In their study of 14 days, they found that emu oil had eliminated all of the inflammation caused by arthritis, joint swelling, and bone abrasion due to lack of cartilage. Furthermore, none of the patients experienced arthritis pain in their joints and bones after 14 days of topical application. The pain caused by the constant friction of bones rubbing together had disappeared.

In the study, at day one, patients showed a 1% improvement;

at day four, a 30% improvement; at day seven, a 50% improvement; at day 11, an 82% improvement; and by day 14, 100% pain reduction.

They also studied the reduction of arthritic swelling. By day one there was a 2% reduction; by day six, 22%; by day 12, 40%; and by day 14, 100%.

Emu oil is not a steroid, and hence does not have the unhappy side effects of cortisone-like agents. These study results represent an exciting option. In addition, it is not a non-steroidal anti-inflammatory drug (NSAID) like aspirin. As such, it does not have the occasionally dangerous side effects that these other agents have (silent gastrointestinal bleeding, reducing blood clotting ability, reducing kidney function).

As mentioned earlier, emu oil is often particularly helpful in cases of knee and shoulder pain. It is also excellent for relief of stiffness and soreness of hands, wrists, fingers, upper neck, back (particularly the middle of the back), ankles, toes, and feet. It can also help muscle spasms of the lower spine, but because deep penetration is required here, emu oil capsules may be a better choice. Also, topically applied emu oil can be helpful in superficial muscle pain of hip soreness and aching. Again, deep penetration is required here to reach arthritic joints. Few topically applied agents would be able to reach the affected area. However, with the use of emu oil you may get superficial relief simply by *relaxing* the muscles. Deeper, more complete relief may be obtained by taking emu oil capsules orally.

In North America, emu oil tends to be used more by alternative medicine practitioners. We are now gradually seeing emu oil increasingly used in more "orthodox" approaches to healing. It's certainly worth a try for any number of health problems and also as a preventative health measure. More and more people are recognizing that it causes no harm. It may be of particular interest to those people who have been through regular medical channels with no success, or those who are unfortunate enough to have side effects from drugs and medications.

People who are already on the blood thinning agent known as *Coumadin (Warfarin)* should take note. Warfarin acts by dramatically reducing blood clotting. It can be very dangerous for people on Warfarin to take an anti-platelet (anti-coagulating) type agent. This is the side-effect of virtually every non-steroidal anti-inflammatory drug such as aspirin, naproxen, ibuprofen, and ketoprofen. Many people on Warfarin prefer not to go on cortisone for any number of reasons—one of these is that it tends to also cause silent bleeding of the stomach. Silent bleeding anytime is of concern, but when you are already on blood thinning agents such as Warfarin, death can be imminent and rapid.

Another group of people for whom emu oil may be particularly useful is diabetics with joint problems—stiffness and soreness. Emu oil can be used very safely in these people, even if kidney problems are present. Unfortunately, NSAIDs can have adverse effects on kidney function. In someone with borderline kidney function such as diabetics, this can be very critical indeed. It is probably very safe for such a person to try emu oil all by itself or cautiously try it with other topical anti-inflammatories. In this way, it may be possible to eventually minimize the amount of NSAIDs put into the body.

How These Arthritis Sufferers Benefited from Emu Oil:

Dr. Bill Code:

Our middle-aged, slightly overweight salesman swears by an emu oil mixture for his recurrent gouty arthritis.

From Monique Barette, Ontario

I have arthritis in the back of my neck and lately, I was in constant pain. It got to the point that I figured I could try emu oil, just in case it would help. To my surprise, the pain almost disappeared after just rubbing the oil on. I keep using it morning and evening. Maybe it won't cure the arthritis, but being pain-free means a lot to me! My husband also suffers from arthritis and he feels the pain relief, too.

From Luella Holman, Ontario

I suffer from occasional sore shoulder, elbow, and arm pain. I purchased some emu oil and it worked on my arm almost immediately. The elbow and shoulder are getting better. I will continue to use this product and have recommended it to my sister for her shoulder pain.

From Eve Tilston-Jones, Manitoba

The emu oil and the emu oil cool rub have really eased the pain in my legs, back, and feet. My hands and nails are just excellent. I have never been able to grow my nails but now they are hard and healthy. I could use some more of the oil and rub whenever possible.

From D. Stabbler, Unity, Saskatchewan

I have been suffering with arthritis for many years. On February 12, 1999, my son purchased emu oil capsules and lotion for me to use on a trial basis. I took two capsules that day and applied the oil on my sore joints. After starting the capsules it was about two weeks before I noticed an improvement in my condition. The lotion that I applied externally on my sore joints worked almost immediately. My feet get sore when the weather changes and when this happens, I add a couple of drops of emu oil to a basin of hot water and soak my feet, and by the time the water cools, the pain has eased.

I would recommend emu oil capsules and emu oil lotion for anyone who is suffering from arthritis or has sore joints. For me, it has given relief from pain. I know it is not a cure, but it definitely helps to ease the pain and discomfort of my arthritis.

Before we wrap up our discussion of arthritis, we need to point out a small but significant difference. There are two main types of arthritis. One is osteoarthritis, which usually involves large weight-bearing joints such as knees and also the end joints on the fingers. This responds quite well to emu oil. The down-side of some non-steroidal anti-inflammatory drugs (the usual medical route, as discussed), is that they actually *reduce* the joint lining's ability to heal itself. This unfortunately causes the joints themselves to wear out more rapidly.

Osteoarthritis, as has been discussed in Chapter 3, is not only a wear and tear illness. More than ever before, we are close to accepting that it is an autoimmune illness. It has a different outline to it than rheumatoid arthritis. Of course, the diseases bear some similarities, the most notable being the fact that there is likely a genetic predisposition toward them.

Rheumatoid arthritis (RA) involves the joints which join the tops of the hands to the fingers, and other joints throughout the body—especially elbows, hips, and feet. These can get some comfort and relief from emu oil, but we are still in far too early a stage to know whether the disease can be reversed in any way. Unfortunately, none of the medications in use today have had any success in reversing RA. The other groups that fit into rheumatoid (rheumatic) diseases include *systemic lupus erythematosis* or *SLE, Reiter's Syndrome, psoriatic arthritis,* and *ankylosing spondylitis.* Supplements which could improve these include vitamin D, calcium, and magnesium, in addition to emu oil.

Soft Tissue Injuries

Soft tissue injury involves repeated use or major weight strain or blow against a portion of the body. Secondary inflammatory response results—the body is trying to heal and recover the area. An example is carpal tunnel syndrome. This occurs right at the wrist on the inside of the arm, (above the palm of the hand). Sufferers experience tingling sensations, particularly in the early morning and sometimes progressing into the day. It's felt to be partly due to a wear and tear or stress recurrence from things such as typing, playing piano, working at a computer keyboard, and so on. It can also be caused by strong, steady vibrations that shake the wrist for long periods (such as using a jackhammer or chainsaw). It's interesting that even though many of these go on to surgery, symptoms often recur after surgery.

Carpal tunnel syndrome is characterized by congestion, swelling, and extra tissue growth in and around the median nerve. This nerve is therefore pinched on its flow through this narrow track. Emu oil is frequently able to penetrate far enough to give some relief. Its anti-inflammatory properties have a positive benefit. Added ingredients such as eucalyptus, wintergreen, or tea tree oil may act synergistically with emu oil's anti-inflammatory effects, further increasing its benefits.

It's also interesting that a number of people respond well to an increase in certain B vitamins along with emu oil. So, there are choices beyond surgery itself in a number of cases. Occasionally, a course of treatment calls for injection of cortisone, but it's much better to try a gentler course. Of course, injection of anything into the skin always presents somewhat of a risk. Introduction of infection into a joint happens at least 1% of the time, and that of course can create a real problem. Why not use emu oil as a carrier rather than an injection? Australian physicians have had good success with this.

That's one prototype of a soft tissue injury. Another would be tennis or golfer's elbow. As with carpal tunnel syndrome, there is a local area of inflammation and irritation due to repeated use or strain. Emu oil on its own can often be very helpful in helping recovery.

Dr. Bill Code:

When I was first looking at emu oil, I had tennis elbow on my left arm (not from tennis, unfortunately, but from digging in the hard clay soil out here on the coast). I put on some emu oil thinking that the effects would be minor, at best. I was quite astounded. Within about 10-15 minutes my elbow was comfortable for the first time in two weeks. Repeated application reduced the inflammatory cycle and soon allowed the tissue to settle down on its own. The emu oil made it possible for me to avoid cortisone injections (and the risk of infection that goes along with any injection).

There are a large number of sports teams, including basketball, football, and hockey, who have used emu oil to help speed recovery and relieve discomfort of localized areas. We see a great many people benefiting from it and speeding their own recovery process. We try to describe it to people as a way to let the body enhance its own recovery process, while at the same time taking away pain and associated problems.

A large number of the testimonials relate to the soft tissue improvement with injuries. In 1997, Doug Atkinson, sports medicine consultant and retired head trainer of the Dallas Mavericks, wrote, "I have personally used emu oil in my training room for the past four years on all injuries that the players of the Dallas Mavericks have incurred. We have had tremendous success in reducing recovery time, thus lowering the number of games missed."

He talks about using emu oil in some of the following cases: kneecap strains and tendinitis, ankle joint soreness, Achilles tendon tendinitis, and entire body soreness.

Alan Hurst of Texas, one of the key people involved in raising emus and later in the processing of the oil, previously worked as a trainer for the Denver Broncos, and is the proud owner of a Super Bowl Ring to prove it. As a trainer, he was quite impressed when he used emu oil in the treatment of football related injuries.

Chiropractors across North America use emu oil in their practice. These clinicians find that emu oil enables them to do a better job of manipulating the spine because the oil reduces muscle spasm. Another advantage is that because emu oil is such an excellent emollient, the client is more comfortable. Patients often get a longer-lasting response to treatment because muscle spasms don't return as rapidly.

Massage therapists are another group frequently very impressed with the benefits emu oil offers. Besides providing the lubrication required to perform the massage, they are also giving their clients the benefits of the oil's anti-inflammatory effects. The penetration ensures the emu oil and any other agents present in the oil reach the site of the inflammation. Individuals who work a great deal with their hands can also experience all the benefits of emu oil, simply by using it as a hand moisturizer or by massaging it into joints or sore areas on the hands daily. Their one concern is that emu oil absorbs so quickly, it may not have enough slip. This is readily solved by mixing with other oils such as almond, coconut, or safflower. This dilution of emu oil is reasonable as most of its properties remain if the mixture is at least 20% emu oil. Of course, more is usually better. The best news, of course, is that there are no unhappy side effects from the use of emu oil.

Chiropractic and massage practitioners often suffer from early osteoarthritis (visible by *Heberden's Nodes)* because they constantly use their hands. A very special but subtle benefit to these practitioners is that the benefits emu oil delivers to the patients is also felt by the practitioners themselves.

If emu oil provides the relief you are looking for when massaged into the affected area, then use it in this manner. If you require still deeper relief, you can also use emu oil gel capsules.

Time is on your side, but give the topical application a few weeks to provide relief. In order to give emu oil capsules a fair trial, use them for at least two to three months.

EPILOGUE

A Final Word
from Dr. Bill Code

Since being diagnosed with multiple sclerosis in August of 1996, I've found a number of things that have helped my illness, stabilizing it and preventing further deterioration. The first of these was in October of that year. Friends of my wife and I wanted to visit, sit down over a cup of tea, and discuss something they felt might help my problems with strength, balance, and stability. It turned out they were talking about insoles which had magnet components to them. Though I was extremely skeptical, the insoles did seem to make a difference. This was my introduction to non-traditional remedies that could help to alleviate the symptoms and severity of my MS. It caused me to start looking at other possibilities that might put me back on the road to health.

In early November of 1996, I called a friend and colleague in Saskatchewan with questions about disability insurance claims. He spontaneously offered to send out a nutritional supplement in capsule form. He felt if I took two of these twice a day, it would make a significant difference for me. He'd already been on them for six months, and felt that they had helped considerably with his rheumatoid arthritis. He sent the product and I began to take two twice a day, as instructed. The product has made a considerable difference with fatigue, level of energy, and mental clarity. You read all about Ambrotose™ in Chapter 6.

This put me on the road to looking at nutrition as a way to help alleviate the symptoms and severity of my MS. How could nutritional supplements make a difference in a long-term chronic illness? I decided two criteria needed to be present in order for me to try something that might make a difference. Number one was that it could not be toxic or harmful to me, my body, or my family. The second criteria was that it had to be relatively inexpensive—most people with a chronic illness have financial struggles. Whenever something satisfies these two criteria, then I'm happy to give it a try.

In the summer of 1996, when I was told I had multiple sclerosis, I had decided to try emu oil. I started with a teaspoon twice a day orally. It tastes much like olive oil. You can take it right off a teaspoon or mix it with vinegar and put it over your salad. Later, I started taking an equivalent amount in capsule form. I have continued this for some four years now. I find it reduces my fatigue. It certainly improves my energy in the morning upon rising, and maybe makes a difference with regard to the recurrence of symptoms. It is now recognized that emu oil, applied topically, can have anti-inflammatory effects in parts of the body other than where the oil was applied.

I knew emu oil was completely safe to take internally, and a considerable number of people were starting to take it either in liquid or capsule form. My best impression of how it works in people is that it has an anti-inflammatory component. Why would this matter in multiple sclerosis? When people get an acute flare-up of multiple sclerosis, it is typically inflammation or swelling of the coatings of the nerves inside the spinal cord and brain. If one can reduce even slightly this swelling and inflammation with an anti-inflammatory, then it makes sense that it would be beneficial to take in the long-term, as long as it did not have major side effects. This anti-inflammatory component is why steroids (like prednisone) are used in short bursts when people have a major flare-up of their multiple sclerosis. I have been fortunate to this point and have not needed to use prednisone, or other steroid medications in short-term bursts. I have continued to take the emu oil and continue to suggest it to people, as it may be part of the factor in reducing the severity and frequency of their recurrences.

I also knew that emu oil contained the essential fatty acids that are needed for human intake and in an acceptable pattern, that is, a ratio somewhere between 10:1 and 4:1 of omega-6 to omega-3. This was another reason to look at something that contained these essential fatty acids: to enhance my nutrition towards stabilizing or, if possible, reversing my chronic illness—multiple sclerosis.

After doing some more research, I found that oils from seeds or animals which originate in cooler climates are healthier. This is because they have higher amounts of the polyunsaturated fatty acids that we need and want. The first of these is of the omega-3 pathway: alpha-linolenic acid; the second from the omega-6 pathway: linoleic acid. These are the only two essential fatty acids that humans need in their diet and, as such, I wanted to optimize my intake of these particular entities. This, then, of course, was the second reason I took the emu oil orally.

In the study of essential fatty acids, I discovered that the respective pathways offered particular benefits, and recognized that omega-3 was the one that the majority of people in North America were short of. In addition, I knew that the omega-3 pathway was very important with regard to recovery and function of not only nerves, but also the lining of nerves in the brain, spinal cord, and peripheral nervous system. This, then, encouraged me to embark on a better and more frequent source of omega-3.

Initially, I used Canadian flax oil, which is very high in

omega-3s and relatively low in omega-6. This seemed important, because we know that excessive omega-6 EFAs, with a corresponding poor balance of omega-3 EFAs, can cause secondary inflammatory problems. For the first several months I used flax oil by itself or along with the emu oil (again, you can take it straight or sprinkle it over salad).

Over time, I learned it was useful to take freshly ground up flax seeds, because this provided the optimal components and minimal potential for rancidity of the oil. It also delivers the benefits of the fiber. The fiber includes lignins, which are recognized to help prevent bowel disease, as well as being a factor in reducing heart disease and atherosclerosis. I had already discovered that the omega-3s are very important in reducing clotting. Therefore, they tend to reduce your risk of heart attack and stroke.

I now take two tablespoons of ground up Canadian flax seeds per day. This might be on hot cereal such as oatmeal or sprinkled on cold cereal. It is quite tasty in either a shake or a smoothie (which is made with fruit juices). Alternatively, it can be added to salad.

In summary, there were two very good reasons to continue with flax seed. The number one reason was that it was very high in omega-3s which would help my balance of omega-3s to omega-6s. The second reason was that the increase of omega-3s would reduce the likelihood for inflammation throughout my body, (for me particularly in the brain and spinal cord—where MS inflammation strikes). In addition, it had the secondary benefit with regard to preventing bowel cancer and reducing the likelihood of developing heart disease. Finally, it is a great fiber and keeps me regular (no constipation).

The next major discovery for me was linking my migraine headaches to food allergies. It is known that 80 per cent of people with multiple sclerosis suffer from migraines. This led me to think about the fact that MS specifically might be linked to food allergies as well. I had been learning more and more about nutrition and how what we eat (and don't eat) affects our overall state of health. You have already read a great deal about my food allergies in the main portion of the text. I feel much healthier and more energetic if I avoid wheat, dairy products, and orange juice. I also rarely get migraine headaches.

My most recent change in diet and supplements was based on the vitamin D data of Dr. Embry (of Calgary) and Dr. Vieth (of Toronto), et al. Their article linking lack of vitamin D to MS was published in the August, 2000 "Annals of Neurology", Vol. 48, pp 271-272. The article was titled "Vitamin D and Seasonal Fluctuations of Gadolinium Enhanced MRI (Magnetic Resonance Imaging) Lesions of Multiple Sclerosis". They described how this special type of MRI shows worsening of MS lesions in people about sixty days after good summer exposure to sun and the resulting vitamin D from it.

Vieth's article (previously referenced) of 1999 outlined the safety of 4,000 IU of vitamin D in supplement form (see Chapter 6). I have been on 4,000 IU of Vitamin D3 for five months now. I now believe I may not have any further exacerbation of my my multiple sclerosis if I stay on my current path.

My hope is my personal journey with chronic illness can help you, your family, or your friends with their own journey. In this way, perhaps they can have "Youth Renewed" the way I have.

Best Regards,

William E. Code

APPENDIX

Scientific Studies, Fatty Acid Analysis, and Testimonials

A t the 1996 11th World Congress of Anaesthesiologists, Dr. Code presented a paper entitled "Non-Opiate Centrally Acting Analgesics". As part of this paper, he introduced to the orthodox medical establishment the concept of emu oil and its anti-inflammatory properties. It seemed the perfect stage to present emu oil, as the emu is native to Australia, the location of the Congress that year.

Emu oil has been used for centuries by Australian aborigines for wound healing and its other medicinal properties. The emu is a fascinating bird—a descendent of the dinosaur and a species virtually unchanged in the past 80 million years. In the search for "new" medicines and nutritional sources, the emu provides us with many of the properties that, as humans, we require in our quest for optimum health.

The emu is unique in its reproductive behaviour and physiology. The birds develop a fat pad, which stores enough nutrition to see the bird through its annual nest-sitting cycle. The male sits the eggs for 52 days. In that time, his temperature drops by 2°C and he doesn't eat, drink, or defecate. Congress delegates heard how this fat pad is replenished and stored annually. This adipose tissue can then be harvested and prepared in such a way so that it still has particular properties on human skin and other animal skin. One of the key properties of emu oil is its ability to penetrate human skin.

In 1996, anaesthesiologists were already well-established on the route of trying to deliver drugs and other agents transdermally (through the skin's surface). Dr. Code was suggesting that this was another way emu oil could be used—in efforts against pain by using its topically carrying capabilities. He also outlined the original patent filed in the U.S. in November, 1991[1] by Australian scientists—so-called Australian "inventors" Peter Ghosh, Michael Whitehouse, Michael Dawson, and A.G. Turner. These scientists originally believed that the polyunsaturated fatty acid was the active component in emu oil. However, their study showed that the active principle seemed to be the yellow components in the oil which possessed this remarkable prophylactic and anti-inflammatory immuno-regulant activity. It also showed an ability to modulate disease once it had already started. So they had sorted this particular yellow component out and talked about it being key.

Dr. Code realized that this was a very new concept for medicine. He expected peer review studies would be forthcoming, and they have continued to turn up in the literature.

"Moisturizing and Cosmetic Properties of Emu Oil: A Double Blind Study", Presented at the AEA National Convention in Nashville, Tennessee, August, 1994, By Alexander Zenstov, M.D., N.S., Indiana University School of Medicine Monica Gaddis, Ph.D., Ball Memorial Hospital Montalvo-Lugo, M.S. and Ball Memorial Hospital

Summary
Cosmetic and moisturizing properties of emu oil were assessed in a double blind clinical study. Emu oil in comparison with mineral oils was found overall to be more cosmetically acceptable ($p<0.05$) and had better skin penetration/permeability ($p<0.05$). Furthermore, it appears that emu oil in comparison with mineral oil has better moisturizing properties, superior texture, and lower incidence of comedogenicity, but probably because of the small sample size these differences were not found to be statistically significant ($p<0.05$). Neither of the oils were found to be irritating to the skin. Finally, emu oil fatty acid composition was studied by gas chromatography and was found to have high concentration of non polar monounsaturated fatty acids which may explain emu oil's ability to penetrate easily through the stratum corneum barrier.

Results showed that emu oil overall ranking and permeability was found to be clearly superior to mineral oil. These differences in skin penetration/permeability and overall ranking were statistically significant ($p<0.05$). It also appears that emu oil texture and moisturizing properties as judged by the participants in the study were also superior to mineral oil, but the differences cannot be considered to be statistically significant (p<0.05). The sample size in this study was small (11). When the partici-pants of the study were asked which of the two oils they liked better, all 11 subjects (100%) stated they liked the emu oil better.

The next study was published in January, 1996. It was published in the *Drug and Cosmetic Industry Journal.* It was an article discussing *Kalaya* oil and cosmetics. *Kalaya* is an aboriginal word for emu, and this was trade-marked in the United States. They admit in the article that it is actually just emu oil. This article was originally written by a Michael F. Holick, Ph.D., M.D. of Boston University Medical Centre and James F. Kinney, M.S., M.B. of San Mar Laboratories.

It started out by saying that the indigenous people of Australia (that is, the aborigines) had appreciated or discovered fortuitously, that the healing and magical power of the oil of the emu was quite useful to them. In fact, when Dr. Code was in Australia, he saw that it was often a major part of their dances, folklore, and culture. Emu oil was shown to be useful any time there was a injury. They would cut off a piece of fat and apply it to the skin for healing, with dramatic benefits. Of course, this was shown to the white man. They also use it for the treatment of muscle and joint disorders.

After that, emu oil was starting to become a little more widely known. The article (in the *Drug and Cosmetic Industry Journal)* summarizes a pilot pre-clinical animal study of oil done at the Boston University Medical Centre. Specifically, Holick and his colleagues were looking at new prod-ucts that would enhance skin and hair growth. They go on to describe the skin as being a complex tissue that contains in its upper layer the epider-mis. This layer produces a very thin layer on the skin, the *stratum corneum.* This is the outer covering that serves as a barrier preventing moisture loss from the skin. It also serves as a barrier to harmful or toxic substances entering the body. We are trying to overcome this "protection" when we use carrying agents such as emu oil or DMSO[2].

Below the epidermis is the dermis, which houses a series of different structures, including the hair follicle. As we age, there are a lot of changes in both the upper and lower levels of the skin *(see figure 8-1).* One major aging change that occurs is dryness. We notice dryness as either roughness, or sca-liness, wrinkling, or laxity (so-called "looseness")—*non-tethered* skin. The majority of these changes occur in the epidermis. There is a loss of epider-mal "fingers" that penetrate into the dermis. You can think of these as little pegs as being like tent pegs that extend from one layer, tethering it to the lower layer. These epidermal "fingers" are called *rete pegs.* They are important because they tether the skin routinely across the surface between the two lay-ers. As they start to disappear, the skin is more mobile. Also, the skin does not get nutrition as well from below and also undergoes a thinning. Holick's study went on to show that emu oil, when compared to corn oil, was much better at returning the "regrowth" of these rete pegs. They noted an improvement in both skin thickness and health occurred with emu oil.

The major changes that occur in the lower base of the skin is that 20% of dermal thickness is lost in older individuals. This accounts for the paper-thin skin of the elderly or chronically ill. There is also a decrease in the amount of elastin fibers, which provide elasticity to the skin, causing the skin to be less resilient. Hence the search for an ideal topical moisturizer that would help aging skin reverse its dryness and scaling by enhancing the ability of the skin's upper layers to retain water. It would be best if this product could also get into the epidermis and stimulate growth cells. This would allow it to enhance the length of the rete pegs or help restart them. Emu oil, they found, could increase skin thickness by 30%.

In their study they used a mouse model. They studied hair growth by histologic (under slides and microscopes) analysis. The hair follicles had an enhanced progression from their resting or sleeping state known as *telogen* to a more active enhanced growth or proliferative state called the *anagen state*. Their conclusion was that the emu oil was able to enhance the growth activity of the skin and also to stimulate resting hair follicles to proliferate and grow. They went on to say that you couldn't directly move from this animal study to humans, but it was very suggestive toward this possibility.

Holick went on to describe previous work by other researchers on the changing composition of the lipid (or oil) types from the different layers of skin (i.e., from the bottom to the top, or from the *dermis* to the *epidermis*). There was an increasing amount of longer chain fatty acids. This is the body taking the two essential fatty acids (EFAs) that we all need (omega-3 and omega-6) and combining them in some particular fashion to make a longer chain fatty acid. What this means is that we don't need to eat that particular longer chain fatty acid as long as we get adequate amounts of the building blocks, i.e., the omega-3 and omega-6 EFAs. It is this shift towards longer chain fatty acids which tends to enhance the hydrophobicity (water held in) as a natural moisture barrier.

In drier and elderly skin, this higher fatty acid composition and secondary decrease in phospholipids permits a larger, more visible stratum corneum. This may be a similar condition to what actually happens in people when they get flaking of skin, commonly known as dandruff. In his article, Holick went on to suggest that the composition of emu oil seemed to be fairly close to the lipid (fat) portion of the skin's stratum corneum. This may be part of the reason emu oil is able to penetrate so well.

He went on to describe that emu oil, when applied to the skin, enhances the skin's ability to withstand the harshness of colder and drier climates. In fact, tests with a group of skiers showed little or no more weathering than normally observed on the face and other exposed skin.

Holick also outlined that when emu oil was used with color-treated hair, hair was more manageable, less brittle, easier to comb and had a much richer, deeper, more natural color. In statements from hairstylists who use emu oil regularly in hair coloring, a few drops of oil per batch of dye produces a much deeper and more rapid uptake of dye into the hair. This also fits with the studies in other animals and repeated observations where injured hair (for example in a horse) will recover more quickly. Also, instead of coming back as white hair (originally *naturally* pigmented), it comes back as original hair, that is, with color, immediately following treatment.

The people in Holick's quoted study went on to say that emu oil works very well in combination with other phospholipids. This would include both the entrapped portion of the liposome (which is a sort of small, manufactured fat globule) and with individual blends of other oils such as palm, sesame, safflower, borage, and coconut-derived phospholipids. Therefore, it is felt that emu oil would be an excellent additive in health and beauty aid treatments. Emu oil provides cosmetic chemists with a unique tool for making hair, skin, daily needs, and other over-the-counter products.

The article goes on to state how one can actually replace or enhance some of the components already in shampoos with emu oil. More particularly, by replacing the ammonium laurel sulfate with emu oil for the rich, silky feel, we probably end up with a more natural, healthier outcome.

An additional paragraph talks about eye care creams. The skin around the eyes is particularly thin and blood supply to it is very good. It very quickly shows changes in allergy or irritation situations. This is always where we swell up first, and also where we have dark circles. This is where we tend to get premature thinning of the skin seen as wrinkles or age lines. It also explains, of course, why people tend to have eye "tucks" or injections of collagen much sooner than anywhere else.

Alpha hydroxy acid, a common ingredient in many of today's over-the-counter skin products, actually causes a degree of chemical burn. Emu oil works superbly well on burns, taking away not only pain but also enhancing healing and recovery of the skin from the chemical burn.

Sunscreen
Emu oil is increasingly being used as a sunscreen protectant in both Australia and in North America. As Holick describes it, he believes the oil

"locks-down" UVA/UVB absorbents more firmly to the skin, and therefore enhances the longevity of the sun protection. Dr. Code suspects that sometime in the near future we will be putting less of the sunscreen protectants on our skin.

The reasons are twofold:

(1) Because of our anxiety of their chemical origin; and

(2) Because sunscreens do not protect against the very serious death-causing skin cancer: malignant melanoma. Be that as it may, Dr. Code has supplied the oil to many friends and clients. They have had a superb recovery from sunburn, sun irritation, even without sunblock.

If you look at the actual ultraviolet protection of the oil all by itself, it's only in the range of 1:2, which is very low on the sunblock scale. It must be working by another mechanism other than blocking the sun. In Chapter 5, we tell you about the fellow who cycled 5,000 miles across Canada in the middle of summer. He rode 8 to 12 hours per day, using no sunscreen whatsoever, did not wear a ball cap, and applied emu oil several times a day. He did not sustain any burn whatsoever and in fact had an even tan. This is an individual who typically would burn out in the sun, but was able to solve, prevent, or calm down the sunburn effects with emu oil alone.

In another comment, Holick describes how emu oil prototypes, when included in skin moisturizing creams and body lotions, completely outscored their placebo counterparts in both providing visible and feel benefits to all skin types. This was particularly evident after repeated hand washings (which removes our body's oils markedly).

Further, emu oil panel testings gave very encouraging results in the daily needs category. These included shower gel, bath oil, and shave cream products, which were examined for extended periods. In both the bath oil and shower gel, the emu oil-containing products were particularly effective in transforming roughened elbow, knee, and heel areas into silky, smooth skin.

The use of shaving cream with emu oil in it, had very pleasing results for both men and women.[3] In all cases of use, the emu oil component appeared to dramatically soften the beard and protect the skin during and after shaving. The occurrence of in-grown beard problems in the African-American panelists was almost completely eliminated after three applications of the shave cream containing emu oil. Dr. Bill Code, too, has found that a small amount of emu oil with his favourite shave gel or cream (you can use any brand) greatly enhances the slip and comfort of shaving. At the same time, it prolongs the life of the blade and enhances the comfort of shaving, both during and after. This has been repeatedly described by both men and women, even in dry, cold climates such as on the Canadian prairies.

Radiation Burns and Chemical Burns from Chemotherapy

A 42-year old gentleman with severe lymphoma had repeated chemothera-py sessions. He was experiencing a large number of mouth ulcers which were very painful. This is not surprising in view of the fact that the cells which are most rapidly dividing, such as the layer of cells inside the mouth, are particularly injured as a result of chemotherapy. He found a very dra-matic improvement with the sores in his mouth with several swishes of emu oil per day. Also, most of the pain disappeared. The emu oil can either be swallowed or spit out, but either way he had dramatic improvement. Subsequent to this, we have suggested it to a number of chemotherapy patients for mouth sores and mouth problems. Fortunately, it also works very well on cold sores (a herpes simplex ulcer). It settles these down very quickly and allows the body to heal. More importantly, it solves the pain component.

Dr. Code has another written testimonial from his father who died at age 79 with lymphoma. He had had a large number of radiation treatments and subsequent radiation burns to his upper neck and face. By applying emu oil he could get 60 to 90 minutes of relief. He used it on repeated occa-sions. This was a bit tricky. Some of the technicians at the facility where he was receiving his treatments said one mustn't apply anything but baby oil. Baby oil is mineral oil. Dr. Code thinks the anxiety comes from the fact that there may be some oils with components of metals or other "focusing" enti-ties which would worsen the burn on some parts of the skin if they were applied prior to radiation therapy. This is a very common and painful prob-lem. Often, the pain requires narcotics (opiates) to treat it. Wouldn't it be better to use a *simple* substance, like emu oil, that worked as well?

The radiation burn success is probably very similar to the response with emu oil on shingles (herpes zoster) infection. Shingles occurs typically later in life. We've already had chicken pox (caused by the same virus) in our childhood. All efforts for developing a chicken pox vaccine have mostly been related to avoiding the extreme pain, which can sometimes be perma-nent, that results from the lesions of herpes zoster as shingles. Again, some-how emu oil seems to take away that pain. This prevents the recurrent pathway buildup of pain within the brain and so-called wind-up within the brain and spinal cord. When this occurs, even once the skin has healed over, pain is sustained and the area is super hypersensitive. The most com-mon site this occurs is one side of the chest, along the breast. People experi-ence so much pain after sustaining shingles that they're unable to tolerate a brassiere or in some cases have difficulty tolerating any clothing over the area at all. It can be so severe and crippling that not a small proportion of people go on to suicide because of its severity. Medical treatment for this usually involves reassurance only. Occasionally, patients will have anaesthesiologists inject epidural painkillers into the local site along that particular nerve or skin branch. Dr. Code's current favourite by far, having tried both of these, is to use emu oil on the site. People are extremely gratified with the results. The prescription solution is a virus killing tablet my mouth. However, even though it often resolves the shingles, it has not been shown to reduce the frequency, incidence, or severity of the pain problem.

Abstract from the American Burn Association, Presented in Chicago, Illinois, March 18-21, 1998: "The Evaluation of Emu Oil in Lubrication and Treatment of Healed Burn Wounds" by M. Penturf, S. O'Banion, and J. Griswold, Study done at Texas Tech University Health Sciences Centre, Lubbock, Texas

Abstract: "Emu oil has been reported to have significant anti-inflammatory effects, and has been used both in cosmetic and therapeutic vehicles. This experiment was conducted to evaluate emu oil as a lubricant and an aid in reducing scar formation in healed burn wounds. Ten patients were evaluated in a randomized double-blind study for a minimum of six months. Patients served as their own control by using bilateral wound areas for application of emu oil and the placebo lubricant on independent sites respectively. Patients were instructed to apply both lotions daily on an as-needed basis. During scheduled out-patient clinic visits, patients' wounds were evaluated by the Vancouver Scar Assessment Scale. Photos were taken on each clinic visit. Patient days ranged from 195 to 385 days before discontinuation. All of the patients were men, ranging from 24 to 62 years of age. For scar assessment, significant differences were noted in pigmentation and pliability ($P>0.02$). There were no differences noted in vascularity and height of the healed wound ($P=0.08$). Pictures were scored by a four-person blinded panel on pigmentation, scar maturation, and general health of the skin. Emu treated areas healed significantly better ($P>0.02$) than control in photo analysis. Statistics were calculated by analysis of variance, means were separated with the F-protected predicted difference test. The results of this pilot study are promising, however additional research is needed to further elucidate any therapeutic qualities of this oil."

Each of the ten people involved put the oil on for an extended period of time. They applied it on both sides of their body, not knowing which was going on which side but consistently using the same one on each side. They weren't assessed personally but the assessment was done on pictures taken at each of their follow-up visits. This was a better way of keeping both caregivers and the person involved blinded. The P>0.02 showed that it was statistically significant 1 out of 50 times. The standard is that it must be P>0.5 to be deemed acceptable. Their results were even better at p>0.2, 19 out of 20 times. They did show significant differences in pigmentation (that is, the return to normal color of the skin) and pliability or softness and flexibility of the skin. So both of these very important features returned more to normal and were confirmed as valid improvement by the people viewing the photographs. It was not quite statistically significant for the vascularity or amount of blood vessels in the area or the height of the healed wound. In reality, it was almost statistically significant, but the sample size of 10 was small. The height of the healed wound is particularly difficult to evaluate in a picture as it does not give you a good 3-D perception. Secondary comments of the people involved were that they felt it was more comfortable when they used the emu oil. Of course they didn't know which oil was which.

This, then is a trial which showed the benefits of emu oil in healed burns. It suggests there are benefits of emu oil on acute burns. We have found emu oil particularly useful and popular among people for heat, cold, or radiation induced burns.

It's important to appreciate that burns are a common cause of death, especially when more than 70% of the body is burned. Though this is improving somewhat today, the problems of pain and death persist. There is a huge adrenaline outpouring of the body because of the pain, and dramatic inflammation in today's burn units. Dr. Code hopes to see the day when emu oil is liberally applied. This would of course necessitate the emu oil being sterile and shown to be successful in a double-blind, controlled trial, but the initial part of this has already happened. Emu oil is now used in individual cases in burn units across North America. Time, we believe, will demonstrate the importance of this particular technique.

The other comment that may bear useful in wound healing is "does emu oil actually provide some of the nutrients right to the skin?" This is quite possible because of emu oil having such good penetration or carrying ability across the skin. Emu oil also contains the two essential fatty acids that we need in skin healing. We've outlined in Chapter 8 how those two essential fatty acids are formed and what their structure is. You learned how they are a very important component of every cell. Fatty acids are actually in the outside layer (wall) of each cell of the body, that is, a protein sandwiched in between a lipid (or fat) bi-layer.

"The Anti-Inflammatory Action of Emu Oils in Rats" by J. M. Snowden and M. W. Whitehouse done at the Department of Medicine, University of Queensland, Princess Alexandra Hospital, Brisbane, Queensland, Australia, Article appeared in *Inflammopharmacology*, 1997; 5: 127-132

Abstract: The anti-inflammatory activities of five different preparations of emu oil, applied topically, have been examined using an experimental polyarthritis in rats. Four of the preparations were found to be active against adjuvant-induced arthritis in rats. The efficacies of the emu oils acting transdermally are compared to that of orally administered ibuprofen (40 mg/kg).

The ongoing discussion within the article is particularly useful. Firstly, it used five different types of emu oil. Two of these were commercially prepared and interestingly enough these are the two that seemed not to have much action. The other mixtures were prepared more carefully, particularly the one mixture which was rendered at a low heat of 40°C and then filtered at 30°C. So now we see a mixture of different types of oils from different types of preparations including inside fat, outside fat (that is the fat in the abdominal cavity vs. the fat under the outside of the skin) and comparisons of these in this particular model. The model is one where the animal is given a mixture by injection which causes a consistent amount of arthritis in a foot. The oil, when it is applied, is actually applied onto the back of the animal. The benefit is assessed by looking at the foot or the front paws. This strongly suggests that the oil is absorbed through the skin and then has an action on the body or is carried by the blood system within the body to the limb and has an action there, reducing the swelling. This is the first paper to show emu oil can be applied on one part of the body and yet works elsewhere.

We need to outline in a little bit more detail how the oils were prepared. The first one was a commercial available preparation from western Australia. The second one was prepared from the fat of emu birds raised by the Department of Agriculture, western Australia. This particular fat had been rendered in a commercial rendering plant and the crude oil did not have any antioxidants added to it. The first oil did have antioxidants added to it. This particular crude oil (No. 2) was stored for about two months before being used and then was filtered again through a cotton wool material. The third emu oil was prepared from the inside of the abdomen or intra-abdominal fat of birds raised, again, by the Department of Agriculture, western Australia. This was prepared by heating in a 650 watt microwave oven on high for about 20 minutes and then filtered through the cotton wool. The fourth oil was prepared from the sub-cutaneous (under the skin) fat of an emu raised in Queensland. This oil was obtained by low temperature (40°C) rendering and clarified by centrifugation at 12,000 cycles for 10 minutes at 30°C. The fifth emu oil was a commercially rendered preparation, again from the fat of birds raised in Queensland. Hence, we have a number of different oils from a number of different geographical and body sites. Perhaps one of the most key items is the method of preparation of the fat into oil.

The other features done within the study included the use of dilutions of olive oil to see if this made a difference, and in fact it did. If there was olive oil in a 1:1 ratio, the oil worked virtually as well as the straight emu oil. However, if the oil was diluted one part emu oil to three parts olive oil, it was not as effective. It is important to note that each of the emu oils or emu oil combinations with olive oils tested included 15% cineole. Cineole is the major turpene taken out of eucalyptus oil and is used as a penetration enhancer. The cineole was tested in combinations with olive oil, alone, or with lard (pig fat) alone, and these, in controlled side experiments, demonstrated no swelling or anti-inflammatory effect.

Other interesting components of this study showed that when the animal was treated with oral ibuprofen at 40mg/kg (which is a good sized dose), that this was equalled in reaction and benefit response to both emu oils 2 and 3 and the benefit or positive response was exceeded by emu oil No 4.

Statistical analysis was by ANOVA T-students tests when significant differences were obtained. The key measurements were done on paw diameter, and it was this that was assessed by the outline of responses or not. The results further demonstrate that not all preparations of emu oil exhibit the same activity. We can only make suggestions as to why this occurred, but certainly the heat that it was rendered at, as well as the source of it, as well as the components of the oil, may all have significant differences. In this study there was benefit from adding the cineole to the oil itself, although this wasn't done in a controlled trial. Certainly there was a disadvantage from adding too much olive oil and perhaps a disadvantage from using the antioxidant. This is still to be determined and warrants further study.

Wound Healing

"Promotion of Second Intention Wound Healing by Emu Oil Lotion:
Comparative Results with Furasin, Polysporin, and Cortisone" by M.J.
Politis, Ph.D., D.V.M. and A. Dmytrowich of Saskatoon, Canada

Dr. Politis outlines how emu oil works particularly well to enhance wound
healing and hence the "second intention wound healing". He states this
because he feels that the immediate application of emu oil lotion, including
emu oil fat, vitamin E, and botanical oil, immediately after creation of full
thickness skin defects delayed wound healing some six days later. He alluded to this perhaps being due to its inflammatory action. However, he goes
on to discuss that following this wait, the administration of the emu oil,
botanical oil, and vitamin E product was delayed for 48 hours. Emu oil
produced a two-fold promotion of wound contraction, epithelialization,
and infiltration of organized granulation tissue.

The testing involved different sites on the back of the animal that were
done with a punch biopsy 6 mm in size. This is quite consistent with what
is used by a dermatologist when taking a skin biopsy. These surgical sites
were observed after the different lotions were applied. Each site was mea-
sured to determine how quickly it healed. As well, they looked at the healing edges under a microscope after the animal was sacrificed. They demonstrated that there was nearly a two-fold promotion of wound contraction,
epiethelialization, and infiltration of organized granulation tissue in the
wounds initially exposed to the emu oil lotion 24 hours postoperatively.
The pure emu oil used in this preparation was seen to promote keratiniza-
tion. It had no significant effect on the wound contraction or the location
of the granulation tissue invasion front. In this particular discussion, he
talks about the emu oil lotion as being emu oil with a combination of vitamin E and a botanical oil carrier. Apparently, in previous studies, it did not
work in the first 24-48 hours. It is interesting if one looks at the literature,
particularly the patent literature. It talks about the enhanced absorption of
emu oil beyond what it ordinarily does, and that it's typically done with the
addition of *cineole*, also known as eucalyptus oil. Alternatively, some people
will add an alcohol to it which tends to enhance absorption. Examples of
this would include ethanol and isopropyl alcohol.

In addition, the emu oil talked about here included both the oil and the
fat in preparation. How was the "pure" emu oil prepared? Could it possibly
have been stripped of some of its ideal properties in its refining steps? This
could include the addition of caustic sodas to neutralize the free fatty acid

fraction of the oil. Sometimes excessively high heat either in the rendering process or in the deodorization process is used. These particular questions are not answered by the article itself, and require clarification.

In discussion of the article, it showed that there was a 55% reduction in wound size in the emu oil lotion group. This was very dramatic. There was a slight slowing of healing relative to the control with the cortisone. This is not surprising because we know that it does slow wound healing. The antibiotic mixture No. 1 was *furazin*, which made minimal reduction in wound size of some 5 to 10%. The other antibiotic, a polysporin, had a 15-20% reduction in wound size.[4]

Wound healing is certainly a complex process, and has a number of phases within it. Wound contraction is a continuous process combining particular cell types and other factors. Chronic administration of anti-inflammatory agents, such as cortisone, if given immediately after injury, has the ability to inhibit the wound healing process. More studies will certainly be required to give a biochemical assessment as to how some of these agents work. The author, Dr. Politis, did go on to say there are several possibilities in how the emu oil might work. His first discussion was how the emu oil lotion may have a cell recovery and wound healing process. He outlined how when the agent is applied to equine hooves and human nails, it promotes growth by 2-3 fold. He states that the emu oil lotion promotes thickening of the epidermal epithelium and studies are now underway to see if the emu oil lotion is effective in tissue culture studies. There has been no data to indicate any unpleasant or cancer-like changes in the skin cells studied to this point. Dr. Politis states that it is possible some of the beneficial effects of emu oil lotion are the result of a synergistic action of emu oil as a trans-cutaneous carrier for molecularly active components in the agent. It is also worth noting that the peroxide levels of extracted emu oil fat (a measure of biochemical degradation) is as high as 30% in some commercial emu oil products, whereas this level is below 2%. This again goes to support some of Dr. Code's earlier contention that maybe the oil used in this particular setting (the "pure" emu oil) had lost some of its valuable properties.

The final summary statement of the author: "In summary, emu oil lotion is a potentially useful agent in the treatment of full-thickness wounds if applied after the inflammatory stages of wound healing." Hence, the initial inflammatory stages in this particular scenario are seen as 24 hours in duration.

"The Effect of Emu Oil on Auricular Inflammation Induced with Croton Oil in Mice" (summary of), Published in the American Journal of Veterinary Research, Vol 60, No. 12, December, 1999, pp 1558-1561 Authors: López, A., Ph.D. & Sims, D.K., et al, from Atlantic Veterinary College, Charlottetown, Prince Edward Island, Canada

This study was supported by National Research Council funds. Dr. Code knows a couple of the people that were involved in the study and has met the two first authors of the study. They're excellent scientists and researchers. The authors wanted to look at the acute anti-inflammatory effects of topically applied emu oil. They did process their own emu oil in their own unique way. He suspects it's not completely dissimilar to some of the ones already listed. Their study was done on 96 mice separated into four groups. A standardized method to start up ear inflammation—50 microlitres of a substance containing Croton Oil dissolved in acetone—was used. Croton Oil is used because it's recognized as an acute cutaneous inflammation produced with minimal discomfort to the animal. Evaluation is done by assessing the degree of inflammation with careful measurement with calipers, or alternately, by weighing the pieces of auricular tissue (that is ear plugs). The effects of the croton oil were transient inflammatory action. This was recognized grossly by a mild hyperemia, which is fluid swelling, with thickening of the ear itself. These changes were particularly apparent when they compared the inflamed ear with the non-inflamed ear. Twenty-four hours later, there was no swelling grossly visible, and there was no sign of any problems as far as necrosis, ulcerations, or discomfort during the study. Their control in the study was porcine oil, which is lard or pig fat. They went on to quote other studies to show that aloe vera preparations had reduced the swelling in a similar model to this and that emu oil was at least as useful and sometimes even more effective in reducing the swelling in this particular case. There was actually some improvement from the porcine oil as well, suggesting that certainly oils do have some anti-inflammatory effects. However, this has never been reported or talked about with lard or pig fat. Dr. Code believes this takes us back to the issue that to some degree healthy animal oils are good for the skin. This, in turn, takes us back to the long-standing concept that bear oil or bear fat was used on injuries, as was goose grease and other agents down through the course of history.

Their final statement was that they were unable to tell how emu oil reduced the swelling—whether this was by diminishing the fluid exudation (permeability edema) or whether it increased the removal or taking away of the fluids by the lymphatic system, or a combination of both mechanisms. Certainly our discussion with regard to eicosanoids suggests that it may well be a diminished fluid exudation that occurs due to the reduction of negative or bad eicosanoids. Of course, the increased blood supply and flow to the area would make a difference with regard to taking away the edema better and/or the supplying of nutrients.

Dr. Code is pleased to be able to summarize different studies from different parts of the world. It is particularly exciting to note the most recent two studies are from Canada. In total, there are two studies from Canada, two from the U.S., and one very important one from Australia. In addition, the Australians have validated emu oil's therapeutic benefits within their health care protocols. This was quite important to permit ethics approval of the first human study by Dr. Zenstof in the U.S. More research need to be done on this very old entity—emu oil—yet very new to most of us.

ASSORTED TESTIMONIALS

My Experience with *Slm3.com*™

I have struggled with my weight since my late teens, always a few pounds overweight. As I progressed into my 30's, the weight seemed to continue to pile on. Never drastically overweight, I was never happy with my weight or the way my clothes fit me.

I suspected my problem was with my liver and gallbladder because of ever-increasing frequency and severity of gallbladder attacks. This, of course, was a function of a lifetime of eating too many trans fats. My diet was always quite good, that is, I didn't eat that much junk food, but obviously it could stand improvement. But in the late fall of 1999, I would have done anything just to stop the gallbladder attacks. That's what got me thinking about the liver cleanse and *Slm3.com* program.

In just two months on the program, while taking the product, I experienced virtually effortless weight loss. It was remarkably freeing to experience a pound lost every few days, knowing how healthy my body was becoming. I was very diligent with the program. I ate no foods considered liver-toxic and made sure that every day I was getting plenty of essential fatty acids. I ground up flax seeds, sunflower seeds, and almonds, and sprinkled this mixture on virtually everything I ate.

I don't have to tell you how gratifying it was to see the pounds melt off. I was doing only minimal exercise at the time—not enough to cause weight loss, and yet I still lost 13 pounds easily. What was so nice about this program was that I was never hungry. I never once counted calories. I never once counted fat grams. Food tasted good. I felt light, energetic. I was thinking so clearly, and was able to concentrate so well on work.

I would recommend this way of eating and the Slm3.com liver cleansing program to anyone. You cannot imagine how good you feel.

— Claudia Tiefisher

Songlines® Emu Oil Testimonials

ACNE

My wife and I have been pleasantly surprised by the wonderful effect of your emu oil on our youngest daughter's acne. She is 14 years old, and a typical teenager with a few facial blemishes that she was very concerned about. Her two older sisters had gone through this phase with standard drugstore remedies, but they didn't seem to be helping Cathy.

When we visited your farm on your open house weekend, we bought a vial of 100% emu oil, and suggested that she use a little bit each night. The next month even our neighbour noticed that her face had dramatically cleared up! Now my other two daughters are using the product for general facial health. Originally it seemed more expensive, but each application uses so little oil that the small container will last for months. They spent a lot more money on cosmetics that didn't help them.

—Victor Brunka, Toronto, Ontario

BURNS

Being an auto mechanic, I was under a vehicle cutting a bolt with a torch. The bolt rolled into the sleeve of my coveralls and stuck to my arm. By the time I crawled out from under the truck, got my coveralls off, the bolt had already burnt into the flesh about a quarter inch. I used emu oil on the burn 3-4 times a day for about a week and to this day it is hard to find the exact spot where the burn was. Our whole family uses emu oil for any little scrape, itch, burn, etc. We cannot say enough good about this oil.

— Doug English, Saskatchewan

CRACKED SKIN

I am a plumber and I work out in extreme cold weather in the winter, with my hands constantly in water. I have tried all types of hand creams and lotions to give relief to my hands, which often get so bad that they crack and bleed. After attending a seminar, my wife purchased some emu oil, and I thought, what the heck, we'll give it a whirl. I am very skeptical about new products, so when I tried the oil, I couldn't believe that it actually worked on my hands. After work, every evening, I apply the oil, more so in the winter than in the summer, and my skin no longer cracks. We always have a supply of it in the house.

— Peggy and Glenn Griffin, Oregon

SHINGLES

I suffered with a severe case of shingles. Not being able to stand the itch and aggravation, and after trying medical and home remedies, I was desperate. My daughter had a sample of emu oil, so I tried it. It truly did help! The emu oil relieved the itch and soreness, and within a week of constant use, my skin returned to normal. Emu oil does work!

— Paul Heglon, Saskatchewan

ECZEMA

My son has a severe case of eczema and needs a prescription every time it flares up. His feet and wrists are bothered the worst, and get so bad that they crack and bleed. It was suggested to us to try emu oil, and to our surprise, within 2 to 3 weeks of using this, his eczema cleared up! Thanks to the emu oil we no longer need to use cortisone, and his eczema is under control. I would recommend anyone to try emu oil. We're glad we did!

— Laurie Renaud, Saskatchewan

CARPAL TUNNEL SYNDROME

Does anyone out there suffer from carpal tunnel syndrome? I do. I have found that rubbing emu oil into both wrists works much, much better to relieve the aching (so that I can sleep at night) than wearing splints and/or taking Relafan constantly. In fact, with all the keyboard "users" in this country, and all the workers' compensation claims being filed because of this growing problem for employers [carpal tunnel syndrome], we need to provide information on the benefits of emu oil to all major businesses in America and their insurance companies who are paying the medical bills for employees who develop this ailment.

— Jane Helt, SandCastle Ranch, U.S.

Composition of Selected Fats (by %)*

Oil or Fat	omega-3 %	omega-6 %	oleic acid %	Saturated Fat %
lard (pig)	0.01	6.7	39.4	48.1
tallow (beef)	1.5	2.3	43.1	40.6
ostrich	1.9	16.0	30.5	40.0
emu (Canadian)	1.7	16.0	53.0	29.0
emu (Texas)	0.3	12.7	42.0	30.0
chicken fat	1.0	20.0	45.0	30.0
olive oil	0.0	8.0	82.0	10.0
flax (Canadian)	57.0	18.0	16.0	9.0
flax (other)	53.3	12.7	20.0	9.5
canola	10.0	24.0	60.0	6.0
soybean	7.0	58.0	23.0	14.0
corn	0.0	59.0	24.0	12.0
sunflower	0.0	66.0	20.0	10.0
cottonseed	1.0	40.0	18.0	31.0
safflower	0.4	75.0	12.0	9.0
grapeseed	0.0	70.0	16.0	10.0
borage	0.0	78.0	—	—
primrose	0.0	81.0	11.0	8.0
walnuts	10.0	53.0	23.0	9.0
almonds	0.01	20.1	65.1	9.6
peanuts	0.0	31.7	49.3	13.8
brazil nuts	0.01	36.0	34.6	24.3

* There are monounsaturates other than oleic,
so total of fats may not add up to 100%.

Chapter Notes

Chapter 1
1 Adapted from *Fats that Heal, Fats that Kill* by Udo Erasmus, Alive Books, Burnaby, B.C., 1993.
2 *Fats that Heal, Fats that Kill* by Udo Erasmus, Alive Books, Burnaby, B.C., 1993
3 Adapted from *Fats that Heal, Fats that Kill* by Udo Erasmus, Alive Books, Burnaby, B.C., 1993.
4 Erasmus, Ibid.
5 *Textbook of Medical Physiology*, 7th Edition, Arthur C. Guyton, M.D., W.B. Saunders Company, 1986.
6 Erasmus, Ibid.
7 Erasmus, Ibid.
8 Erasmus, Ibid.
9 Erasmus, Ibid.
10 Erasmus, Ibid.
11 Erasmus, Ibid.
12 Erasmus, Ibid.
13 Erasmus, Ibid.
14 Erasmus, Ibid.
15 *New England Journal of Medicine*, "Trans Fatty Acids and Coronary Heart Disease", 2000, Volume 340, #25, pp 1994-1998. This report states that trans fatty acids are twice as bad as saturated fatty acids.

Chapter 2
1 Flax seeds are indigestible in the sense that you cannot obtain essential fatty acids from eating them whole. However, consuming the whole seed, ground up, provides excellent nutrition in the form of insoluble fiber.
2 *Prescription for Natural Healing*, James F. Balch, M.D. and Phyllis A. Balch, 1997 by Avery Publishing Group
3 *American Heart Association Fat and Cholesterol Counter* 1991

Chapter 3
1 If you have trouble digesting this food, you may be wise to consider eliminating it from your diet. If you consider the stone age diet, (which is what we are genetically designed for) beans and peas would necessarily be excluded because stone age peoples lacked the fire to cook this food and therefore would not have consumed it. Some experts theorize that only foods that can be eaten raw should be included in the "ultimate" diet.

2 This would have had to be whole grain brown rice, with all the benefit of the rice bran, etc.

3 *Apple Cider Vinegar Health System* by Paul C. Bragg, N.D., Ph.D. and Patricia Bragg, Ph.D., Health Science, 1989

4 *Kidney Disorders* by Martha J. Miller, Chelsea House Publishers, 1992

5 *Clinical Psychiatry News* 26(5): 34, 1998

6 *The Journal of the American Medical Association,* October 22, 1997; 278:1327-1332

7 With proper attention to allergen-causing foods (orange juice, wheat and dairy), Dr. Code's irrirable bowel syndrome doesn't bother him very often anymore. It is interesting to note, however, that IBS and its symptoms were a forerunner to his being diagnosed with MS. It is his theory that food allergies and the resulting autoimmunity in a condition such as IBS were the "early" stages of MS.

8 *Apple Cider Vinegar Health System* by Paul C. Bragg, N.D., Ph.D. and Patricia Bragg, Ph.D., Health Science, 1989

Chapter 4

1 It has to be said that almost all alcohol companies openly and aggressively promote responsible drinking. When we look at the ills caused in society by this activity, however, it would be easier to simply not drink and avoid the circumstances that inevitably seem to follow.

2 *The Liver Cleansing Diet* by Dr. Sandra Cabot, M.D., 1996 SCB International

3 An excellent liver cleansing product is *Slm3.com*™ by Deliteful Foods, available in health food stores. It contains all the essential ingredients to facilitate optimal liver function and resulting natural weight loss. See also weight loss testimonials from the use of this product and adherence to this program in the Testimonials appendix on page 251.

Chapter 5

1 Dr. Code is in no way suggesting that it is safe or desirable to use emu oil instead of sunscreens having a recognized sun protection factor (SPF) of at least 15 or more.

Chapter 6

1 *The 120 Year Diet* by Roy Walford, M.D., Four Walls Eight Windows Publishing, New York, NY, 2000

2 Walford, ibid.

3 *Biochemical and Physiological Aspects of Human Nutrition,* by Martha H.

Stipanuk, Ph.D., W.B. Saunders Company, 2000

4 Vieth, R. 1999 "Vitamin D Supplementation, 25-hydroxy-vitamin D concentrations and safety" *Am. J. Clin. Nutr.,* Vol 69, p. 842-850

5 Stipanuk, ibid.

6 *Real Age* by Michael F. Roizen, M.D., HarperCollins, New York, NY, 1999

7 *Encyclopedia of Nutritional Supplements* by Michael T. Murray, N.D., Prima Publishing, 1996

8 *Advanced Nutrition & Human Metabolism,* by Groff, J.L., Gropper, S.S.: Wadsworth, 3rd Edition, 1999

9 Roizen, Ibid, p. 158

10 *The Secrets to Great Health,* by Dr. Jonn Matsen, ND, Goodwin Books, North Vancouver, B.C., 1998

11 Groff, J.L., ibid.

12 *Nutrition Action Healthletter*, May 1998

13 Murray, ibid.

14 *Nutrients in Food* by Elizabeth Hands, Lippincott, Williams & Wilkins, 2000

15 Cordain, L., et al "Dietary Modulation of Immune Function in Rheumatoid Arthritis", *British Journal of Nutrition*

16 Quoted in the October, 1999 and June, 2000 issues of the *University of California at Berkeley Wellness Letter*

17 Stipanuk, ibid.

18 Stipanuk, ibid.

19 Stipanuk, ibid.

20 Groff, ibid.

21 Stipanuk, ibid.

22 Roizen, Ibid, pg. 171

Chapter 8

1 *How Your Body Works,* by Susan L. Engel-Arieli, M.D., Ziff-Davis Press 1994

2 *Human Anatomy and Physiology* by John W. Hole, Mr., Wm. C. Brown Publishers, 1990

3 Glygcosaminoglycans, present in high amounts in glucosamine, are popularly used to combat arthritis because of their ability to attract and hold water. This water cushions joints.

4 Please see the Scientific Studies appendix for a full report of this study.

Chapter 9
1 See study summary beginning in Scientific Studies.

Scientific Studies Notes
1 Approved July, 1995, patent No. 5431294
2 dimethyl sulfoxide: a liquid industrial solvent, not approved for human use; for veterinary use.
3 This result was recorded by both African-American and Asian participants.
4 This study of Politis, M.J. (of Saskatoon, Canada) and A. Dmytrowich is published in *Plastic & Reconstructive Surgery* Dec, 1998, Vol. 102, #7 pp 2404-2407.

Glossary

ADHD – Attention Deficiency Hyperactivity Disorder: a condition characterized by inability to concentrate, focus or sit still. Often medicated with *Ritalin*. Has been linked to a deficiency in omega-3 fatty acids.

aerobic exercise – any physical activity that makes the heart and lungs work harder to meet the muscles'need for oxygen.

alveoli – tiny air sacs of the lungs where carbon dioxide leaves the blood and oxygen is taken on by the blood.

anaerobic exercise – oxygen is used by the muscles faster than it can be supplied by the bloodstream.

anaesthesiologist – a doctor of medicine graduate who studies five years to specialize in caring for people during surgery, intensive care and pain management (e.g., labour, surgical and trauma pain).

anaphylaxis – a sudden and rapid swelling of the body, especially breathing and airway. Usually an allergic response.

anthocyanins – any of several water-soluble nitrogenous pigments which contribute to the red, blue, or violet colors in some plants (e.g. cherries, grapes, plums). Powerful antioxidants.

antioxidants – substances (e.g. vitamins C and E) that remove potentially damaging oxidizing agents in a living organism.

atherosclerotic plaque – fatty or waxy substance that builds up in arteries leading to atherosclerosis (hardening of the arteries).

autoimmune disorder – one of a large group of diseases marked by a change of the immune system of the body. The body's defense system is turned against the body itself, causing chronic and often deadly diseases; many of these disorders have now been linked to allergies.

B. bifidus – a beneficial bacteria that lives in the gut.

bad fats (damaging) –*trans* (hydrogenated or partially hydrogenated) dietary fats, especially when consumed in excess.

beta carotene – a precursor of vitamin A found in carrots, tomatoes, etc., and converted in the body to vitamin A.

blood sugar – the amount of glucose in the blood.

cholesterol – a sterol found in most body tissues including the blood, where high concentrations promote arteriosclerosis. Some cholesterol is needed by the body, however, for brain function and the manufacture of certain hormones, particularly sex hormones.

cis fatty acid – a fatty acid configuration where the hydrogen atoms of the carbon atoms involved in the double bond are on the same side of the molecule, causing the molecule to bend or kink.

cold pressed – oils extracted from seeds or nuts without the use of *hexane*, and done at low temperatures.

collagen – the main protein substance of the body; responsible for the form and shape of most tissues (except bone and cartilage).

comedogenic (non-comedogenic) – acne causing (non-acne causing).

complex carbohydrate – sugar molecules strung together to form longer, more complex chains. Complex carbohydrates include starch and fiber.

cosmeceutical – a cross between a "cosmetic" and a "pharmaceutical"—a cosmetic product that is expected to have some therapeutic or active beneficial component(s).

delta-5-desaturase – an enzyme in the human body that converts components of fatty acids to "bad" eicosanoids. This enzyme is not present in the skin.

dermatitis – any mild or moderate inflammation of the skin causing rash and/or itchiness.

dermis – the thick layer of living tissue below the epidermis (skin).

desensitize – slowly and gradually reduce response, e.g., allergy to bee stings; or fear of heights.

disease – an unhealthy condition of the body or mind; illness, sickness.

dis-ease – an alternative medical practitioner's term for a state of the body that can be termed to be in "*dis*"-ease.

diverticuli – tiny pouch-like sacs that develop in the colon, becoming inflamed when matter becomes lodged in them.

duodenum – first part of small intestine, after the stomach.

eicosanoids – hormone-like substances that regulate blood pressure, clotting, immune response, inflammation response and other body functions; formed from omega-6 and omega-3 fatty acids.

emollient – a substance that softens tissues, especially the skin and mucous membranes.

emulsify – to mix a liquid into another liquid, making a suspension that has globules of fat.

emulsion – a mix of two liquids, made so that small droplets are formed, as oil and water.

epidermis – the outer cellular layer of the skin.

Epstein-Barr virus – a DNA herpesvirus which causes infectious mononucleosis and is associated with certain cancers, e.g. Burkitt's lymphoma.

essential fatty acids – several varieties of fatty acids that must be eaten because the body cannot manufacture them. Essential to brain function, manufacture of enzymes and for the integrity of the cell wall.

fiber – the indigestible portion of the diet consisting of various plant cell-wall materials, that passes through the body largely unchanged.

fibroblasts – cells producing collagen fibers in connective tissue.

flu (influenza) – contagious virus infection causing fever, severe aching, weakness, and coughing.

free radicals – a molecular fragment with a single unpaired electron which, wanting to be paired, steals electrons from other pairs.

glucagon – a polypeptide hormone formed in the pancreas, which aids the breakdown of glycogen to glucose in the liver.

glucose – a simple sugar containing six carbon atoms, which is an important energy source.

glutathione – a crystalline, water-soluble peptide of glutamic acid, cysteine and glycine.

glycogen – a polysaccharide serving as a store of carbohydrates, and yielding glucose on hydrolysis.

glycoproteins – any of a group of compounds consisting of a protein combined with a carbohydrate.

Heberden's nodes – an abnormal enlargement of bone or cartilage in a joint of a finger (usually the tip or distal joint).

Hexane – a chemical used to extract oil from seeds and nuts.

high carbohydrate, low fat diet – a diet that, because it is low in fat, is supposed to be good for weight loss.

homocysteine – an substance that is converted from methionine, an amino acid.

hydrogenation – the addition of hydrogen to an edible oil to convert it into a saturated fat, usually solid at room temperature.

hypercholesterolemia – a condition characterized by an excess of cholesterol in the bloodstream.

hyperlipidemias – any condition characterized by an excess of fats in the bloodstream.

hyperthyroidism – overactivity of the thyroid gland, resulting in a rapid heartbeat and an increased rate of metabolism.

hypothyroidism – decreased activity of the thyroid gland.

indigestion – difficulty in digesting food; pain or discomfort caused by this.

innocuous – harmless, non-toxic.

insulin – a polypeptide hormone produced in the pancreas by the islets of Langerhans, which regulates the amount on glucose in the blood, and the lack of which causes diabetes.

Islets (or Islands) of Langerhans – small parts or globules of special cells (millions of them) within the pancreas. These islets secrete insulin and glucagon.

lactic acid – a carboxylic acid formed in the muscle tissues from glucose and glycogen during strenuous exercise.

lactobacillus acidophilus – a good bacteria present in the gut.

life process – a stage of life such as growth, puberty and menopause.

liposomes – a microscopic spherical sac consisting of a lipid envelope enclosing fluid; often used in medicine to deliver drugs to target tissues in the body.

liver – large, lobed, glandular organ in the abdomen, responsible for metabolizing fats, detoxifying and neutralizing foreign and toxic substances.

melatonin – a hormone produced in the body and which helps us sleep.

metabolism – the life process of cell, which takes place in the mitochondria of the cell.

monosaccharides – a sugar that cannot be hydrolized to simpler carbohydrates of smaller carbon content. Glucose and fructose are examples.

monounsaturated fatty acids – fatty acids whose molecules contain one double bond in its carbon chain (contains one point of unsaturation).

motility – description of movement, e.g., food along intestinal tract.

muscle – tissue consisting of elongated cells (muscle fibers) containing fibrils that are highly contractile.

non-food – any "food" that contains no life energy – few vitamins, minerals, fiber or anything beneficial to sustain health; usually processed and packaged.

pancreas – a digestive organ/gland in the body which manufactures digestive enzymes as well as insulin and glucagon, hormones vital to control of blood sugar levels in the body.

peristaltic – kneading or massaging, as in the action of the esophagus when pushing food down toward the stomach.

phospholipid – any of a group of fatty compounds, composed of phosphoric esters, present in living cells (e.g. lecithin).

phytates – compounds present in some foods that affect absorption of certain vitamins or minerals.

phytochemicals – plant chemicals beneficial to human health when ingested. Some are known to prevent cancer.

polyunsaturated fatty acids – any fatty acid molecule which contains more than one double bond in its carbon chain.

potassium hydroxide – an ingredient often used in skin care products; known to be a skin and eye irritant.

precursor – raw material before body the makes it into something else, e.g., glucose into glucosamine or beta carotene into vitamin A.

proanthocyanins –colored plant pigments which act as powerful antioxidants in the body.

proinflammatory – any substance which tends to enhance, or increase, the inflammatory process.

prostaglandins – one of a group of fatty acid derivatives, originally identified in human prostate secretions but now known to be present in all tissues. Different prostaglandins often have opposite actions.

protein – one of a large group of substances that are important in the structure and function of all living organisms.

quercetin – a bioflavonoid.

saturated fatty acids – a fatty acid which contains no double bonds; present in almost all fats to some degree, but highest in animal fats.

serotonin – a neurotransmitter (carries messages between nerve cells); works opposite to melatonin; serotonin is produced in response to increasing daylight to help you get out of bed in the morning.

smooth muscle – involuntary muscle of all internal organs; usually in the form of tubes or sheets, which may be several layers in thickness

stratum corneum – the outermost layer of skin, where dead skin cells are sloughed off.

sustained release – a process like *timed release*, e.g. when consuming carbohydrates high in fiber, the sugars (carbohydrates) are released more slowly than if the food consumed had no fiber.

synergy – when the sum of two or more substances, working together, is greater, or more beneficial, than if each of those substances were working separately.

trans fats – a fat that has been changed from its original form through either hydrogenation, heating or other type of action; usually refers to poly or monounsaturated fatty acids that have had their double bonds broken and hydrogen added.

triglycerides – a molecule of fat or oil consisting of 3 fatty acid molecules hooked to a glycerol backbone.

vesicles – a small, sac, cyst or cavity, especially one filled with fluid.

whole foods – any food that hasn't undergone changes by manufacturing or processing; a food that is as close as possible to its original, natural form.

Bibliography

101 Most Asked Nutrition Questions, by Patricia Chuey, M.Sc., R.D., Eating for Energy, Vancouver, B.C., 1999

21st Century Natural Medicine, by Dr. Douglas Lobay, N.D., Apple Communications, Kelowna, B.C., 1992

Advanced Nutrition & Human Metabolism, by Groff, J.L. and Gropper, S.S.: Wadsworth, 3rd Edition, 1999

American Heart Association Fat and Cholesterol Counter 1991

Apple Cider Vinegar Health System, by Paul C. Bragg, N.D., Ph.D. and Patricia Bragg, Ph.D., Health Science, 1989

Basic Chemistry, G. William Daub and Willliam S. Seese, Prentice Hall, Upper Saddle River, NJ, 1996

Beauty to Die For, by Judi Vance, ProMotion Publishing, 1998

Biochemical and Physiological Aspects of Human Nutrition, by Martha H. Stipanuk, Ph.D., W.B. Saunders Company, 2000

Bragg Toxicless Diet, Paul C. Bragg, N.D., Ph.D., Health Science Publications, 1973

Chemistry of the Body, by Janet E. Garden and Robert A. Richardson, John Wiley & Sons Canada Limited, 1985

Cider Vinegar, by Cyril Scott and John Lust, N.D., Benedict Lust Publications, 1992

Eating Well for Optimum Health, by Andrew Weil, M.D., Alfred A. Knopf, New York, NY, 2000

Emu Farmer's Handbook, by Maria Minnaar, Nyoni Publishing Co, Groveton, Texas, 1998

Emu Oil: Reexamining A Natural Remedy with Today's Technology, compiled by Sherrie Schatz and Sheree Lewis, published by Emu Today & Tomorrow, LLC, Nardin, OK, 1996

Encyclopedia of Nutritional Supplements, by Michael T. Murray, N.D., Prima Health Publishing, Rocklin, CA, 1996

Essential Fatty Acids in Health & Disease, by Edward N. Siguel, M.D., Ph.D., Nutrek Press, Brookline, MA, 1994

Everywoman's Medical Handbook, by Dr. Miriam Stoppard, Ballantine Books, New York, NY, 1988

Facts on File Dictionary of Biology, Edited by Robert Hine, Checkmark Books, New York, NY, 1999

Fats that Heal, Fats that Kill, by Udo Erasmus, Alive Books, Burnaby, B.C., 1993

How Your Body Works, by Susan L. Engel-Arieli, M.D., Ziff-Davis Press 1994

Human Anatomy and Physiology, by John W. Hole, Wm. C. Brown Publishers, 1990

Human Anatomy, by Kent M. Van De Graaff, Wm C. Brown Publishers, 1992

Kidney Disorders, by Martha J. Miller, Chelsea House Publishers, 1992

Liver Cleansing Diet, by Dr. Sandra Cabot, M.D., 1996 SCB International

Mosby Medical Encyclopedia, by Glanze, W.D. and Anderson, Kenneth N. and Anderson, Lois E., Penguin Group, Toronto, ON, 1992

Nutrients in Food, by Elizabeth Hands, Lippincott, Williams & Wilkins, 2000

Nutrition, Chemistry & Biology, by Julian E. Spallholz, Prentice-Hall, Englewood Cliffs, NJ, 1988

Nutrition Bible, by Jean Anderson, M.S. and Barbara Deskins, Ph.D., R.D., William Morrow & Company, New York, NY, 1995

Omega Diet, by Artemis P. Simopoulos, M.D. and Jo Robinson, HarperCollins, New York, NY, 1999

Omega Plan, by Artemis P. Simopoulos, M.D. and Jo Robinson, HarperCollins, New York, NY, 1998

Personal Nutrition, by Marie A. Boyle and Eleanor Ross Whitney, West Pub Co., New York, NY, 1989

Prescription for Natural Healing, James F. Balch, M.D. and Phyllis A. Balch, 1997 by Avery Publishing Group

Professional's Handbook of Complimentary & Alternative Medicines, Charles W. Fetrow, PharmD and Juan R. Avila, PharmD, Springhouse Corporation, Springhouse, Pennsylvania, 1999

Random House Health and Medicine Dictionary, Random House Publishers, New York, NY, 1992

Real Age, by Michael F. Roizen, M.D., HarperCollins, New York, NY, 1999

Secrets to Great Health, by Dr. Jonn Matsen, ND, Goodwin Books,, North Vancouver, B.C., 1998

Take Charge of Your Body, by Dr. Carolyn deMarco, The Well Woman Press, 1996

Textbook of Medical Physiology, 7th Edition, Arthur C. Guyton, M.D., W.B. Saunders Company, 1986

The 120 Year Diet, by Roy Walford, M.D., Four Walls Eight Windows Publishing, New York, NY, 2000

The Complete Canadian Health Guide, University of Toronto Faculty of Medicine, Key Porter Books, 1993

Whole Way to Allergy Relief & Prevention, by Jacqueline Krohn, M.D., Hartley & Marks, Point Roberts, WA & Vancouver, B.C., 1996

Index